**American
Red Cross**

CAT FIRST AID

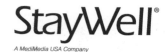

StayWell®

A MediMedia USA Company

Dedication

This book and DVD set is dedicated to the feline friends that have been our partners and loyal companions for thousands of years. May we continue always to bring out the best in one another.

Note to Our Readers

No matter how sweet their disposition under normal circumstances, *all* cats have the instinct to scratch and bite when frightened, injured or threatened. So **always protect yourself by muzzling and/or restraining your cat with a towel** before providing first aid, especially if what you need to do might cause more pain. If you cannot safely capture and restrain an injured animal, call your local animal control officer for assistance.

There is a very low risk of transmitting infection between humans and cats. However, the use of nonlatex, disposable gloves is recommended when treating cat wounds to keep the wound clean. This is not absolutely necessary so do not delay providing care to your cat if gloves are not available.

The editors agreed that "it" is not an appropriate pronoun for a cat. So to avoid awkward and wordy "he or she" and "him or her" sentence constructions, we alternated the gender reference throughout the text.

When you see this DVD icon in the book margins ⊚, it means the skill is demonstrated or the topic is covered in greater detail on the enclosed DVD.

Printing/Binding by RR Donnelly, Spanish Fork

StayWell
780 Township Line Rd.
Yardley, PA 19067

Library of Congress Cataloging-in-Publication Data

Cat first aid.
    p. cm. — (Be Red Cross ready safety series ; v. 3)
  ISBN-13: 978-1-58480-402-4
  1. Cats—Diseases—Treatment. 2. Cats—Wounds and injuries—Treatment. 3. Cats—Health. 4. First aid for animals. 5. Veterinary emergencies. I. American Red Cross.
  SF985.C2955 2008
  636.8'08960252—dc22

                            2008035086

ISBN 978-1-58480-402-4
08 09 10 9 8 7 6 5 4 3 2 1

About the American Red Cross

Mission of the American Red Cross

The American Red Cross, a humanitarian organization led by volunteers and guided by its Congressional Charter and the Fundamental Principles of the International Red Cross Movement, will provide relief to victims of disaster and help people prevent, prepare for and respond to emergencies.

The American Red Cross helps people prevent, prepare for and respond to emergencies. Last year, almost a million volunteers and 35,000 employees helped victims of almost 75,000 disasters; taught lifesaving skills to millions; and helped U.S. service members separated from their families stay connected. Almost 4 million people gave blood through the Red Cross, the largest supplier of blood and blood products in the United States. The American Red Cross is part of the International Red Cross and Red Crescent Movement. An average of 91 cents of every dollar the Red Cross spends is invested in humanitarian services and programs. The Red Cross is not a government agency; it relies on donations of time, money, and blood to do its work.

Fundamental Principles of the International Red Cross and Red Crescent Movement

Humanity

Impartiality

Neutrality

Independence

Voluntary Service

Unity

Universality

Acknowledgments

This *Cat First Aid* book and DVD set was developed and produced through the combined efforts of the American Red Cross and StayWell. Without the commitment to excellence of both employees and volunteers, this product could not have been created.

The American Red Cross and StayWell thank: Alternatives NY, Advertising and Design Agency; Pat Brown, St. Louis Area Chapter; Christine McLaughlin, writer; David Spagnolo, cover photographer; Todd Trice, photographer; Main Line Animal Rescue; and Vickie Wooters, Wooters Dog Training for their contributions to the production of this book and DVD.

The American Red Cross and StayWell also thank the following individual who provided expert review of the materials and support for *Cat First Aid*:

Deborah C. Mandell, VMD, DACVECC
Staff Veterinarian, Emergency Medicine
Adjunct Assistant Professor
Section of Critical Care
Matthew J. Ryan Veterinary Hospital of the University of Pennsylvania
Philadelphia, Pennsylvania

Table of Contents

CHAPTER 6: FIRST AID REFERENCE GUIDE

Table of Contents

Table of Contents

Foreword

One of my fondest, early-childhood memories is of my two cats Puffy and Cocoa. It was cute to see how, when they napped together, the gentle, lady-like Puffy would wrap her leg protectively around Cocoa, our loud and boisterous Siamese. After Puffy died, Cocoa moped around and seemed very sad. He finally cheered up after we got a Dachshund puppy.

Cocoa spent many happy years with me and lived to the ripe old age of 21! My next cat, Sasha, accompanied me through veterinary school, internship and residency. So, I know first hand how important your cat is to you and your family. That's why I am very proud to work with the American Red Cross to bring you *Cat First Aid*.

During my years as an emergency and critical care veterinarian, I have learned that cats will try to hide signs of illness until a disease is very advanced. So I hope this book will serve not only as a handy first aid reference guide, but will also help you learn what is normal for your cat so you can recognize subtle cues of health problems sooner. Seeking veterinary care early will give your cat the best chance for successful treatment.

Cats are amazing; their personalities are as unique as our own. They will let you know when they want affection and when they want to play. Having a cat may reduce feelings of stress and loneliness. And several studies have shown a correlation between pet ownership and improved health. So, next time you need to unwind, just have a cat lie in your lap and listen to him purr as you gently stroke his fur.

Wishing you many happy and healthy years with your feline friend,

Deborah C. Mandell, VMD Diplomate ACVECC

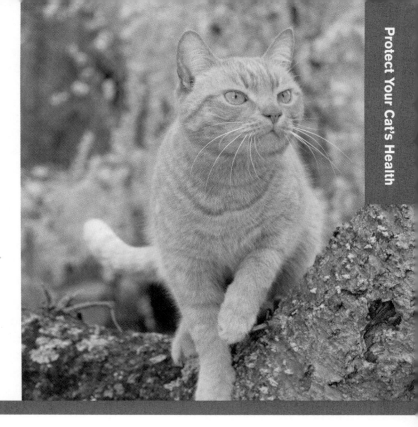

1

Protect Your Cat's Health

You bought this book because you are obviously concerned about your cat's welfare and want to be prepared for health emergencies that might arise from sudden illness or injury. The same responsibility that inspires you to help your cat when something goes wrong is equally important in ensuring his life is full of good health and happiness. In return for your time, love and care, your furry friend will enrich your life immeasurably.

Keep Your Cat Healthy

Take Your Pet to a Vet

Regardless of how you acquire your cat or what age he is when you get him, be sure to schedule a health check-up with a veterinarian as soon as possible. He or she will make sure your cat receives all the necessary vaccinations and has the proper tests and prevention medications for heartworm and other parasites.

It is crucial to keep your pet's vaccinations up to date. Kittens require a series of inoculations; ask the veterinarian about an appropriate schedule. Take your adult cat to the veterinarian at least yearly.

Your pet's veterinarian is also a great source of advice. Do not hesitate to discuss any behavior concerns you may have.

Provide Good Daily Care

Proper diet and exercise will help you keep your pet lively and trim throughout her life. And be sure your pet is groomed regularly.

Proper Diet. Feed your cat the proper amount and type of food. Choose a well-balanced, name-brand or premium-brand cat food that is appropriate for your cat's stage of life. Avoid generic foods because they may not be held to the same rigorous quality standards. Consult your veterinarian about an appropriate diet for your cat.

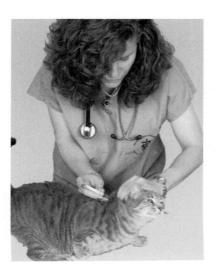

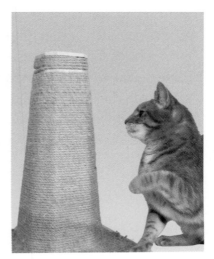

Keep Your Cat Healthy

Always provide your pet with an adequate supply of clean water and change it frequently.

Regular Exercise. Exercise is important for cats. Encourage your cat to move and play by tapping into his natural hunting drive with cat-specific toys like balls, feathers on rods and laser pointers. Also, a scratching post may not only spare your favorite recliner, but give your cat a safe place where he can stretch and work his shoulders.

Safe, Comfortable Environment. All cats should be indoor companions, living as members of a family. Cats that live outdoors can become aggressive and dangerous. It is best not to allow your cat to roam outside. Your pet might be hit by a car, be injured by other animals, eat poisonous materials, bite someone, contract and spread diseases (including rabies), get lost or stolen or become a victim of abuse. But if your cat does go outside, make sure her identification is affixed to her collar and that her collar is the type that snaps off if it gets caught (sold in pet stores).

Cats like to hide and nap in warm, cozy places. Unfortunately, sometimes this can be very dangerous, and the consequences can be devastating. For example, cats have been known to hide inside chimneys, clothes dryers, sofa beds, trash compactors and on top of a car's warm engine in cold weather. So always be sure to check these places before using them, and keep your cat away from them while in use. Make a habit of banging on your car hood a few times before starting the engine.

Put a sticker on the front door or front window of your home to alert others that a pet is in your home in the event of an emergency. You can order a free pet rescue sticker from the American Society for the Prevention of Cruelty to Animals at *www.aspca.org*.

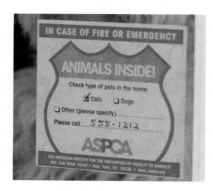

tips

PESTICIDE DOs AND DON'Ts

Do—

1. Read all labels and follow directions carefully.
2. Make sure insecticides are safe to use in combination if using more than one product, such as—
   - A flea collar and a dip.
   - More than one kind of flea insecticide.
   - Professional exterminator chemicals used around the home.
3. Talk to your veterinarian about how to treat your pet and her environment safely.

Don't—

1. Use a product more frequently, in higher concentrations or in a larger quantity than directed on the label.
2. Use a product for an age group or animal not specifically mentioned on the label.
3. Use products labeled for small dogs on cats.
4. Use pesticides on extremely young or old, sick or pregnant cats.

Good Grooming. Brush and comb your cat's coat regularly to keep it healthy and free of matted hair. Begin doing so when your cat is young so he gets used to this, especially if you have a long-haired cat, as they are prone to developing matted fur.

Ask the veterinarian to show you how to safely clip your cat's nails and care for his ears. Regular grooming will also help you detect skin problems and parasites such as fleas and ticks early. (See pages 93–94 for information on tick removal.)

Cats with fleas often bite and scratch themselves excessively. If you notice this behavior, look for evidence of fleas. (See Fleas, page 89.) Talk to your veterinarian about how to treat your pet and your pet's environment safely.

Spaying and Neutering

Pet overpopulation is like a disease—it kills millions of cats each year. But there is a cure: spaying (for females) or neutering (for males). This cure also has health and behavioral benefits for your pet. The American Veterinary Medical

Association and others agree it is safe to spay or neuter most kittens as early as 8 weeks of age.

When performed early, spaying can prevent breast cancer (mammary tumors). Spaying at any age eliminates the risk of uterine infections and uterine or ovarian cancer.

Pets that are spayed or neutered are usually better, more affectionate companions, and neither you nor your pet needs to suffer through the physical and behavioral problems associated with heat cycles. Spayed or neutered pets are less likely to roam, spray or mark territory or be aggressive.

NOTE: Spayed or neutered cats do not automatically become fat and lazy.

ID—Your Lost Pet's Ticket Home

Even though your pet should live indoors and remain under your supervision when outside, cats should wear collars (purchase one that has a quick-release buckle) and up-to-date identification at all times.

If your cat becomes lost, a tag with your name, address and phone number can help reunite you and your pet. But regardless of the type of ID on your cat, search for your lost pet immediately. Contact local animal shelters and pet stores, put up signs and call all surrounding veterinarians.

If all else fails, visit these lost pet Web sites:

- Lost Pet SOS: *www.lostpetsos.org*
- Find That Pet: *www.findthatpet.com*

How to ID Your Pet
Follow these tips to make sure your cat has proper ID at all times:

- Affix license and/or rabies tags to your cat's collar as required by state or local law.
- Add a tag with essential medical information for cats with medical problems.
- Attach a temporary tag when traveling with your cat, with a contact name and phone number of where you'll be staying.

- Consider having a microchip implanted under your cat's skin by a veterinarian or animal shelter. The microchip—about the size of a grain of rice—contains a code that a scanner can detect and read. Always register your pet's microchip with the national database.
- For back-up ID, have an ID number permanently tattooed on your pet and register the number with a recognized national organization such as Tatoo-A-Pet (*www.tattoo-a-pet.com*), which can be reached by phone at 1-800-TATTOOS (1-800-828-8667) or by e-mail at *info@tattoo-a-pet.com*.

Traveling with Your Pet

Some cats will be happier if allowed to accompany their owners when they travel. However, you must always balance this need against his overall health and safety. If you are moving to a new area, of course you will take your pet with you. You simply need to consider the best and safest mode of travel for your cat. However, if you're thinking about taking your cat on vacation with you, you must consider your pet's health, whether your pet likes to travel, where you'll be staying, the time of year, your options if you don't take your cat and whether taking your cat on a vacation is really in his best interest.

If traveling abroad, be aware that some countries have requirements that can take up to 6 to 8 months to complete, so start planning as early as possible.

Have your cat examined by your veterinarian before any trip. Get any required legal travel documents (contact the airline as well); make sure vaccinations are up to date and get any medications your pet might need. Medications used specifically for travel should be given to your pet on a trial basis several days before you leave to make sure your pet doesn't suffer adverse effects.

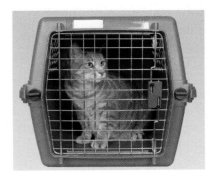

Choose a Good Cat Carrier
A cat carrier is an essential item to have at home. There are hard-plastic carriers and soft-material carriers. A sturdy one may be safer in the event of an accident.

In the Car
When riding in the car—

- Your cat should be in a crate or carrier.
- Your cat should never ride in the front passenger seat, especially one that is airbag equipped.
- Never let your cat out of the car without proper restraint.
- On a long trip, take your pet's travel kit. (See What to Pack for Your Pet, page 8.) Keep a supply of water in the car.
- Never leave your pet alone in a parked car, not even for a few moments; she will be vulnerable to heat distress or theft.

On a Plane
Although thousands of pets fly on airlines without problems, there are risks. Follow these tips:

- Don't fly your cat unless it's absolutely necessary.

- If you must take your cat when you fly, make travel arrangements well in advance, and ask about all regulations, including any quarantine requirements at your destination.
- You may be able to arrange to carry him onboard with you.
- If your pet must travel in the cargo area—
  - Use a direct flight.
  - Travel on the same flight as your pet.
  - Ask to watch your pet being loaded and unloaded.
  - When you board, notify the captain and at least one flight attendant that your pet is in the cargo hold.

If you choose to leave your pet behind while you go on vacation, be sure whoever is caring for him has your vacation phone number, complete feeding and care instructions and the phone number of your veterinarian. It is also a good idea to tell your veterinarian who will be caring for your pet and what your wishes are for veterinary care in case of emergency while you're gone.

What to Pack for Your Pet
Here are some essentials to take when you travel with your pet or if you must evacuate with your pet in a disaster:

- Medications and medical records
- Food and bowls
- First aid kit
- Bedding
- Leash, collar and tags
- Grooming supplies
- Current pet photo that includes you (in case your pet gets lost)
- A favorite toy or two
- A sturdy, well-ventilated carrier
- Litter and litter box

For more information on what to pack in case of a disaster, see Be Prepared for Disaster, page 17.

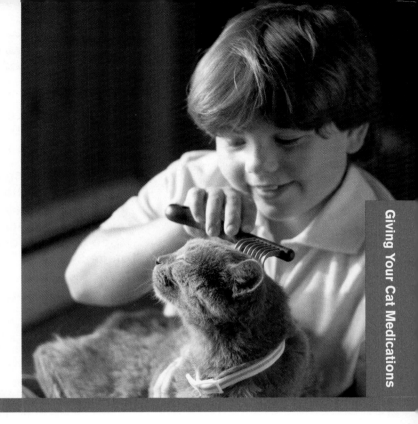

2

Giving Your Cat Medications

Giving Your Cat Medications

It is not a simple task to give your cat medicine, especially pills, and you'll probably have to do it at some point in her life. But following the steps below will help ensure your cat is on her way back to good health. It's important to remember never to attempt to give medications by mouth to an animal that is lying down, unconscious, vomiting, having trouble breathing, having a seizure or acting aggressively.

Administering Eye Medications
Technique

1. Rest the side of the hand that you will use to administer the medication on the bone above your cat's upper eyelid. This will help prevent poking the medication tube into the eye if you are jostled.
2. Tilt the head backward slightly with the palm of your other hand under the chin supporting the head.
3. With this same hand, pull up on the upper eyelid with your thumb.
4. Place drops or ointment directly in the eye with enough distance to ensure the tip of the dispenser does not touch the eye.

NOTE: Wrapping a cat up in a towel so that only the head shows may help you avoid getting scratched. (See Capture Techniques, page 26.)

Administering Ear Medications
Technique

1. Stand on the same side of the animal as the ear you will be treating or behind the cat.
2. Place the drops or ointment in the middle of the ear opening.
3. Rub or massage the base of the ear to allow the medication to drop down into the deeper portions of the ear.

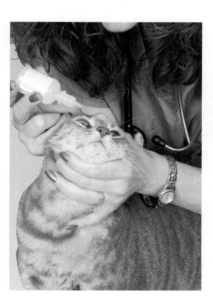

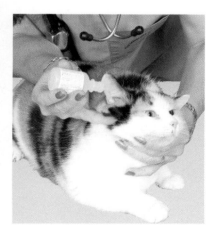

Liquids

For many people, giving liquid medication to a pet is easier than giving pills. Keep a baby dosing syringe or eyedropper (both with measurements marked), which can be found in pharmacies or in the baby section of grocery stores, in your pet first aid kit (see Pet First Aid Kit, page 16).

Here are some common conversions you may find helpful for correct dosing:

- 1 milliliter (ml) = 1 cc
- 5 cc = 1 teaspoon
- 15 cc = 1 tablespoon

Technique

1. Place the end of the eye-dropper or syringe on one side your cat's mouth, just behind the pointy canine teeth where the teeth are shortest and flattest.

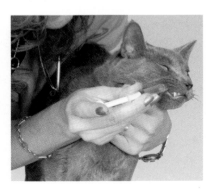

2. Gently position the dropper above the lower teeth, or in the pouch between the gums and lower teeth. (Placing the medicine over the teeth will result in less spitting of the medicine than placing it in the pouch.)
3. Slowly administer the medication, giving it no faster than the animal can swallow.

IMPORTANT: Never give your cat any medications unless they are prescribed by a veterinarian.

Pills and Capsules

Technique

1. With one hand, hold your cat's upper jaw toward the ceiling by taking hold of the snout and gently point-ing it upward. This will cause the lower jaw to drop slightly.
2. With the other hand, gently pull down on the very front-most part of the lower jaw.
3. Place the tablet in the cen-ter of the back of the tongue, as far back into the mouth as you safely can.

Giving Your Cat Medications

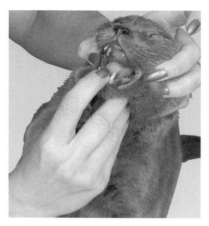

4. Hold the mouth closed once you have given the pill until your pet swallows or licks his nose. Sometimes gently blowing on the nose or rubbing the throat will cause the animal to swallow.

If you prefer, you can try to hide the pill in food, but you must ensure your cat does not eat the morsel and spit out the pill. If your cat is vomiting or has diarrhea, hiding medication in food is not a good idea because it may make the condition worse.

There are also commercial pill "guns" available. These plastic tubes hold the pill and allow you to place it in the back of the throat without putting your hands in the animal's mouth.

Topical Ointments and Creams

Compared with administering pills, ointments and creams are a walk in the park. While wearing disposable, nonlatex gloves, apply the medication in a thin layer. However, the most important thing to remember is to keep your cat from licking the ointment, as it will lessen its effectiveness and might even give her an upset stomach. You might consider putting an Elizabethan collar on your cat to prevent her from licking the medication. Or, depending on where the wound is, you might also consider putting a baby t-shirt on her to cover the affected area.

Elizabethan Collars (E-Collars)

These collars are designed for function, not fashion. They're extremely helpful in keeping your cat from aggravating a wound, biting sutures, or licking off ointments and creams. Your cat may act a little cranky at first and may bang into walls and furniture due to lack of peripheral vision, but it's only temporary, and he'll eventually forgive you, especially after he feels better. You can

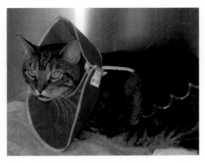

purchase an Elizabethan collar from any pet supply store or from your veterinarian.

Adverse Reactions From Human Food and Medicines

Cats should never be given human food or medicines designed for humans unless prescribed by the veterinarian. Your cat's digestive system, metabolism and nutritional needs are quite different from yours. This means certain foods, medicines and other substances that are fine for you could seriously harm or even kill your pet. In addition, most things that are not healthy for you to eat, such as spoiled food, raw eggs or fish and excessive amounts of sugary and fatty foods, are not healthy for your cat either.

Here is a partial list of foods and medicines to keep away from your cat. Consult with your veteri-narian for a more specific list of foods that are harmful to your cat.

Foods
- Alcoholic beverages (all types, including beer)
- Avocado
- Bones from chicken, fish (and other meat bones a chewing cat can break apart or splinter) – these can cause choking, get stuck in the esophagus or stomach or puncture internal organs.
- Chives
- Chocolate and cocoa (all forms)
- Coffee and other caffeinated beverages (all forms)
- Garlic
- Macadamia nuts
- Milk
- Mushrooms
- Onions, onion powder
- Raisins and grapes
- Salt
- Xylitol sweetened products (typically found in sugar-free gum)
- Yeast dough

Medicines
Even small doses of some human medications can be lethal to your pet. The human dosage is typically too high for a cat and may cause toxic side

effects. Also, cats may metabolize medications differently than humans do, so any dose may be toxic! Some of the major medicines that cause adverse and possibly fatal reactions include:

- Allergy medications, which can cause neurological or cardiovascular symptoms, depending on the drug.
- Antidepressants.
- Anticancer drugs.
- Cold remedies, which can cause neurological or cardiovascular symptoms, depending on the drug.
- Diet pills.
- Nonsteroidal anti-inflammatory drugs (NSAIDs), like ibuprofen (Motrin®, Advil®), naproxen (Aleve®) and aspirin, which can lead to major, life-threatening kidney failure, gastrointestinal bleeding or liver failure.
- Pain killers, including acetaminophen (Tylenol®), which can cause brown gums, a swollen face and difficulty breathing. (These are caused by *methemoglobinemia*, a condition in which the red blood cells are not able to carry oxygen. Just one acetaminophen tablet can kill a cat.)
- Prescription drugs, which can cause a variety of

effects depending on the drug.
- Vitamins (particularly those that contain iron).

In addition, many plants and household products are poisonous to your pet. For example, lilies, and other common household plants, are extremely toxic to cats. For more information, visit the American Society for the Prevention of Cruelty to Animals (ASPCA) Web site at *www.aspca.org* and scroll down to "Animal Poison Control" in the Expert Advice menu on the left.

What to Look For

If you suspect your cat has ingested a drug inadvertently, always look for neurological signs (depression, seizures, hyper-excitability), gastrointestinal signs (vomiting, diarrhea), shock and respiratory distress (see Poisoning, page 95). Call your veterinarian or the ASPCA National Animal Poison Control Center at 888-426-4435 immediately. There is a charge for the consultation. In critical cases, the center will do as many follow-up calls as necessary and will contact your veterinarian at your request.

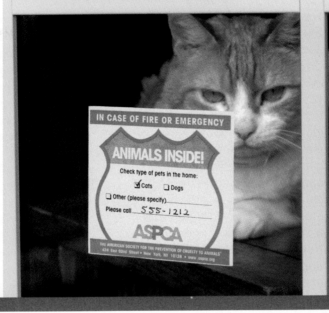

IN CASE OF FIRE OR EMERGENCY

ANIMALS INSIDE!

Check type of pets in the home:

☑ Cats ☐ Dogs

☐ Other (please specify)_____

Please call _555-1212_

ASPCA

THE AMERICAN SOCIETY FOR THE PREVENTION OF CRUELTY TO ANIMALS
424 East 92nd Street • New York, NY 10128 • www.aspca.org

3

Be Prepared

In any type of emergency, having supplies nearby before you need them and knowing how to respond can reduce panic and increase the chance of a positive outcome. This is especially true during a regional disaster when help might be delayed and normal supply chains could be cut off. If an evacuation was ordered, would you be ready to pick up and go at a moment's notice, assured that you have everything you need for your family, including what you need for your pet? Gather the items listed in this section to complete your cat's first aid and emergency supplies kits. For more information about emergency preparedness for your family, visit *www.redcross.org* and click on *Be Red Cross Ready*.

Pet First Aid Kit

Every cat owner should have some basic first aid supplies on hand. If your pet has special medical conditions, ask your veterinarian what additional items you should include. Check your kit periodically to replace expired medicines and replenish used supplies. The pet first aid kit can be stored in a small, sturdy box. Consider carrying a smaller version in your car. Remember to keep all medications and medical supplies out of the reach of young children and pets.

A pet first aid kit should include:

- ☐ Absorbent compresses (sometimes called gauze sponges) in assorted sizes
- ☐ Adhesive tape (hypoallergenic)
- ☐ Antibiotic ointment (triple, available at pharmacies)
- ☐ Blanket (emergency or "space" blanket)
- ☐ *Cat First Aid* book
- ☐ Clean cloth
- ☐ Cold compress
- ☐ Credit card (expired, to scrape away stingers)
- ☐ Epsom salts (to make saline solution)
- ☐ Gloves (disposable, nonlatex)
- ☐ Glucose paste or corn syrup (if your pet is diabetic or has a history of low blood sugar)
- ☐ Grooming clippers
- ☐ Hydrogen peroxide, 3 percent (check expiration date)
- ☐ List of emergency telephone numbers, including your pet's veterinarian, an after-hours emergency veterinary hospital and the American Society for the Prevention of Cruelty to Animals' Animal Poison Control Center (888-426-4435)
- ☐ Muzzle (size that fits your pet)
- ☐ Nail clippers appropriate for your cat's nails
- ☐ Nylon leash (at least one)
- ☐ Penlight
- ☐ Petroleum jelly
- ☐ Rectal thermometer (non-mercury/nonglass)
- ☐ Roll cohesive wrap, 3-inch width (stretches and clings to itself)
- ☐ Roll gauze, 2-inch width, cotton
- ☐ Rubbing alcohol (isopropyl)
- ☐ Scissors, small, with blunt end (bandage scissors)
- ☐ Sterile eye lubricant (available at pharmacies)
- ☐ Sterile eye wash (saline, available at pharmacies)
- ☐ Sterile gauze pads, non-adherent (assorted sizes)
- ☐ Sterile, water-based lubricant (such as KY® Jelly) that

washes off easily (to keep fur away from a wound you are treating)
- ☐ Styptic powder (to stop bleeding from broken nails, available at pet stores)
- ☐ Syringe (baby dose size)
- ☐ Towel
- ☐ Tweezers

Be Prepared for Disaster

A disaster can strike any time and anywhere. It is important to know if earthquakes, floods, tornados or severe weather can affect your area, and whether you live in a special hazard area, like a floodplain, wildfire or hurricane-prone area. If you must evacuate in a disaster, use the recommended evacuation routes. Some areas can be dangerous, so avoid shortcuts. In the case of any evacuation, LEAVE EARLY to avoid heavy traffic or gridlock.

It's equally important to be aware that "natural disasters" aren't the only emergencies you need to be prepared for. Fire, acts of terrorism and other human-caused disasters, such as a hazardous material spill, could require a prompt response.

Get a Kit

You should assemble an emergency supplies kit ahead of time for everyone in your household, including your pet. Keep everything in sturdy containers (duffel bags, covered plastic storage containers, etc.) that can be carried easily. The kit for your cat should include:

- Pet identification (see below for more information)
- A pet first aid kit, including this book, and any medications your pet is taking
- Medical records stored in a waterproof container; include vaccination records, information on your pet's medical conditions, veterinarian's name and phone number and a list of any other special concerns
- Food and water for each pet: a 3-day supply for an evacuation and a 2-week supply for the home, including a manual can opener, if needed, for canned food
- Food and water bowls
- Bedding/blankets and toys to help reduce stress and provide comfort
- Leash, harness and carrier to transport your pet safely and to ensure your pet

Be Prepared

cannot escape (The carrier should be large enough for the cat to stand comfortably, turn around and lie down.)
- Litter box and litter
- Garbage bags, quart-size storage bags, newspapers, paper towels and bleach to make a sanitizing solution for cleaning up pet waste

Pet Identification Is Extremely Important! Your cat should wear current identification on his collar at all times. In case of a disaster, include an additional temporary tag that lists your out-of-area emergency contact phone numbers. It's also a good idea to have a microchip implanted in your pet beforehand, in case the collar and/or tags fall off (see How to ID Your Pet, page 5). Be sure to include photos of your pet taken with you to prove your ownership and to help find your pet if he becomes lost.

Make a Plan
Even if you don't live in a floodplain, near an earthquake fault line, in wildfire country or in a coastal area, it's crucial to think about how you will cope. And remember, if you and your family need to evacuate, so does your pet.

Make a List of Important Phone Numbers. At the top of your emergency preparedness to-do list should be to create a list of important phone numbers. These should include people and organizations in your area, outside of your area and in a different state that you can rely on in the event of a disaster, including your family and friends; pet-friendly hotels; veterinarians/emergency veterinary hospitals; boarding facilities; and, as a last resort, a list of local and remote animal shelters.

Remember that most human emergency shelters will not allow animals, except service dogs, to stay there. Also understand that if you have more than one pet, you might have to house them separately. Thus, it is very important to determine ahead of time where you will take your pet in an emergency.

Be Informed
Depending on the type of disaster, you may need to stay at home or follow an order to evacuate. Plan for both possibilities. Listen to the radio and TV, and check the Internet for up-to-date information and promptly

follow the authorities' instructions. For more information on how to prepare, visit *www.ready.gov* or call 1-800-BE-READY.

IMPORTANT: At the first sign of an emergency, locate your cat and confine her to her carrier so you can leave with her quickly. Be sure to check her favorite hiding spots because that is where she will probably go if she is frightened. Do not wait until the last minute to gather your supplies. Have your emergency supply kit ready to go.

Evacuating With Pets. Call ahead to confirm emergency shelter arrangements for both your family and your pet, whether you're staying together or separately. Be sure your pet and her carrier have up-to-date identification and contact information, including the phone number of your temporary shelter and its location.

If you do evacuate, keep your pet with you or know the designated emergency location where you will take your pet. Animals left inside a home can escape if the home is damaged by storms. Animals left to fend for themselves outside are likely to become victims of exposure, starvation, predators, contaminated food or water or accidents. Leaving cats outside during a disaster is a death sentence.

Staying Home. If you are at home during a storm, identify a safe area of your home where you can stay with your pet. Remember to keep your cat in a carrier, and make sure he is wearing identification. Be sure to have your other emergency supplies handy (see Get a Kit, page 17).

If You're Not Home When Disaster Strikes. Make arrangements in advance with a trusted neighbor who has a copy of your house key. Ask your neighbor to take your pet and meet you at a specified location if a disaster strikes when you're not at home and an evacuation order is issued. Be sure that person is comfortable with your pet and knows where he is likely to be, as well as where your disaster supplies are kept. In addition, have all your contact phone numbers readily available for your neighbor.

Be Prepared

Returning Home After the Disaster. Your home could be a very different place when the disaster is over. So wait until authorities say it is safe for you and your cat to return. Once you do, don't allow your cat to roam loose throughout your home. Familiar landmarks and smells might be gone, and she will probably become disoriented.

For a few days, keep your cat confined to one room inside the house or in her carrier. Try to establish a calming environment and get her back into her normal routines as soon as possible, and be patient with her if she has some stress-induced behavioral problems afterwards. If these persist, or if your pet seems to have health problems, talk to your veterinarian.

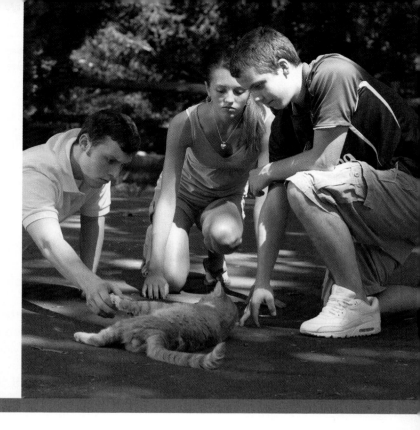

4

How to Know if It's a Medical Emergency

The best way to recognize and respond to an emergency is to know what is normal for your cat and to know how to recognize an emergency. However, if you are unsure about a situation, always call your veterinarian. Many conditions have a better prognosis if caught early. Another important thing to know is that cats compensate very well for most disease processes, which means that by the time your pet begins showing signs of illness, he may already be in an advanced stage of disease. So take him to a veterinarian as soon as possible.

Know What's Normal

It will be easier to recognize what is abnormal for your pet if you first become familiar with what is normal. Observe how your cat breathes, eats, drinks, walks, urinates and defecates so you will be sensitive to changes that might signal problems.

Check the Scene

Before approaching an injured cat, look around for potential hazards that may still exist and could potentially harm you. For example, if an animal has been struck by a car, make sure there are no other cars approaching before running into the street; or if your cat is in a fight, don't get between the two animals or you might become the next victim.

Check the Cat

Make an initial evaluation that should be completed in about 1 minute. Do the following:

- **Situation.** Quickly observe the animal's body; posture; presence of blood, urine, feces or vomit; breathing pattern; and sounds and other materials (possible poisons around the cat).

- **Airway.** Is it open? If not, see Airway, page 32.
- **Breathing.** Is the animal breathing? If not, see Breathing, page 32.
- **Bleeding.** If the animal is bleeding, see Bleeding, page 45.
- **Circulation.** Is there a heartbeat and a pulse? If not, see Circulation, page 33.
- **Mucous membrane color.** See Observe Your Cat's Mucous Membrane Color, page 24.
- **Capillary refill time.** See Capillary Refill Time, page 25.
- **Level of consciousness.** Is the animal alert, awake, seizuring, disoriented, hyperactive, depressed or unconscious? If the animal is seizuring, see Seizures, page 101.

Always have the telephone numbers of your veterinarian, 24-hour veterinary emergency hospital, American Society for the Prevention of Cruelty to Animals' Animal Poison Control Center (888-426-4435) and animal shelter or animal care and control agency readily available!

Heart Rate and Pulse

You can feel your cat's heartbeat at about the point where the left elbow touches the chest (about the fifth rib). Lay your cat down on her right side. But, if it's easier, allow her to stand.

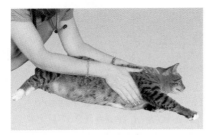

1. Gently bend the left front leg at the elbow and bring it back to where it touches the chest.
2. Place your hand or a stethoscope (available at most pharmacies) over this area to feel or hear and count heartbeats.

You can feel your cat's pulse by lightly touching your middle and index fingers to the inner thigh as follows:

1. Lay your cat down on either side.
2. Gently lift her upper hind leg away from the lower hind leg.
3. Place your two fingers as high up as possible on the inside of either leg, just where the leg meets the body wall.

4. Feel for a recess in the middle of the leg approximately half way between the front and back; this recess is where the blood vessels run and where you will find the pulse.
5. You can also try this with your cat standing up.

NOTE: Remember to use a light touch; if you press too hard, you will not feel the pulse.

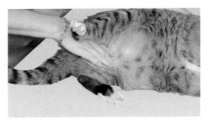

Breathing Rate

1. Your cat can either stand or lie down.
2. Watch your pet and count the number of times that the chest rises and falls in 1 minute.

In an emergency, if you are not sure if your pet is breathing, try one of these techniques:

- Hold a cotton ball or tissue just in front of the nostrils and see if it moves
- Hold a mirror up to your pet's nose and look for condensation

Is It an Emergency?

Respiratory Pattern. When a cat inhales normally, the chest should expand. If the abdomen expands instead of the chest, that could indicate a problem. Exhaling should be an easy process with no work involved. If your pet is breathing through his mouth, open-mouth breathing, makes gasping sounds when breathing or is not breathing, this is an emergency; see Cardiopulmonary Resuscitation, page 32.

NOTE: Cats do not normally pant unless they are frightened or in distress. Cats should not pant for more than a few minutes at a time. If panting appears to go on longer, treat it as an emergency.

How to Take Your Cat's Temperature
1. See Restraint Techniques, page 28.
2. Use a digital thermometer, found in any drug store.
3. Lubricate the thermometer with a water-based lubricant or petroleum jelly.
4. Insert the tip of the thermometer into the rectum (just beneath the tail).
5. Leave the thermometer inserted until it beeps.
6. Remove and read the number.

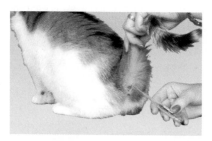

IMPORTANT: A temperature lower than 100° F or greater than 104° F is an emergency; call your veterinarian at once.

What's Normal?
Heart, pulse and breathing rates and body temperatures outside these ranges could signal an emergency:

- Normal heart rate: 160 to 220 beats per minute
- Normal breathing rate: 20 to 30 breaths per minute
- Normal body temperature: 100°–102.5° F

Observe Your Cat's Mucous Membrane Color
The color of your cat's mucous membranes (gums and inner eyelids) can help you determine if enough oxygen and

blood are flowing to all of his tissues. To check the color of the mucous membranes, lift your cat's upper or lower lip and observe the color of his gums or inner lip.

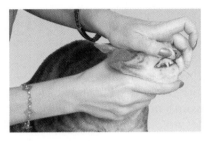

- If your cat has black (pigmented) mucous membranes, place your thumb on the skin just under the lower eyelid and gently pull down to observe the inner eyelid membrane color. It should be pink, which means the tissues are receiving enough oxygen.
- If your cat's mucous membranes are blue, pale yellow, cherry red, white, brick red or brown, this is an emergency. Call the veterinarian immediately.

Capillary Refill Time

Observing how soon the gums or inner lips return to their normal pink color after you press on them is a quick way to know if your cat's blood circulation is normal.

1. After checking the mucous membrane color, press lightly on the gums or inner lip.
2. Observe the color as it turns white and then pink again. The pink color should return after 1 or 2 seconds.
3. Call your veterinarian at once if the pink color returns in less than 1 second or more than 3 seconds. This is an emergency.

How to Approach, Capture and Restrain a Cat

Always approach a sick or injured cat slowly and cautiously. Even your own sweet kitty might strike out if frightened or in pain. Observe her posture and expressions—especially her face, ears, tail, fur and body. Listen to the sounds she's making.

As you approach, allow the animal to smell the back of your hand. Never make quick or jerky movements or loud sounds. Allow the cat to see what you are doing and

Is It an Emergency?

watch her reactions carefully. Always speak in a soft, soothing tone to an injured or sick animal.

Body Language Warning Signs

Any of these behaviors may indicate the cat is inclined to bite. Do not attempt treatment on any cat with any of these warning signs:

- Crouching with ears flattened to the head
- Salivating or spitting
- Small pupils, but they become enlarged as the cat becomes more frightened
- Arching its back with tail up
- Hair standing up
- Hissing

Also, do not attempt to treat a cat that appears to walk on its toes with the head and tail held down, hair partially standing up, ears up and pointed so they open on the sides, whiskers turned forward and claws out.

If you cannot safely handle an animal, call your local animal shelter or animal care and control agency. You can't help an animal if you get hurt yourself. While waiting for assistance to arrive, you can

do other things to help, such as diverting traffic if an animal has been hit by a car and is still in the street, or keeping other people and animals away from the injured animal.

Capture Techniques

If you determine that it is safe to capture a cat, let him know where you are and move slowly and calmly. Speak to the cat in a quiet, soothing voice and try these techniques.

Towel or Blanket. You can sometimes capture a cat by dropping a towel or blanket over her.

1. First observe the cat's position so you don't put your hands near her mouth.

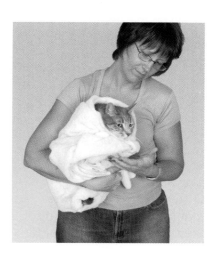

2. Drop a large towel or blanket from above and behind the cat.
3. Grasp the scuff of her neck so she cannot turn around and bite your hand through the towel.
4. Transfer the cat to a sturdy box or carrier.

Boxes. Cats will often crawl into boxes for comfort; you can use the box to transport the cat or to help you administer treatment.

1. If the cat goes into a plastic carrier that can come apart, simply remove the top of the carrier.
2. Drop a towel over the cat.

Gloves. While you might think wearing thick work gloves will help you safely handle a cat, they will cause you to lose dexterity, and some cats can bite and scratch through most glove material. While you cannot catch any diseases from your vaccinated cat through contact with body fluids, you may want to consider wearing nonlatex, disposable gloves when treating wounds to prevent the spread of infection.

Muzzle. You can purchase a cat muzzle at pet stores and

veterinary hospitals and through pet catalogs. This should be part of your pet first aid kit (see Pet First Aid Kit, page 16).

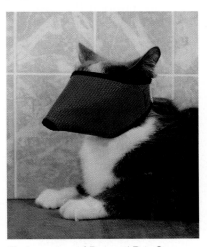

Photo courtesy of Proguard Pets Company.

IMPORTANT: All hurt, sick or frightened animals may be inclined to bite, so they should be muzzled before any care is attempted.

But in some situations, muzzling may be dangerous to the animal; this danger must be weighed against the risk of human injury. It may be dangerous to muzzle an animal that is—

• Having difficulty breathing.
• Coughing.
• Vomiting.

Is It an Emergency?

NOTE: No muzzle is fool-proof, so don't be lulled into a false sense of security while using one. Many pets can get out of a muzzle, especially if it is not fitted correctly.

Some animals will resist being muzzled and might become aggressive. In this case, do not attempt to muzzle the cat or treat him yourself. Take the animal to your veterinarian or seek help from your local animal shelter or animal care and control agency.

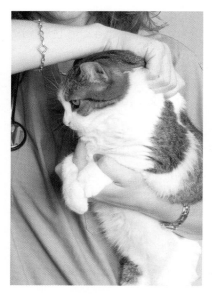

Restraint Techniques

Laying a Cat on His Side.
1. Stand alongside and face the standing cat.
2. Lay him on his side.
3. Hold the legs that are on the table or floor (the down legs).
4. You may have to hold the legs with one hand and grasp the loose skin behind the cat's neck (the scruff) and hold it firmly with the other hand.

Scruff.
1. Grasp the loose skin behind the cat's neck with one hand.
2. Support the cat's body with your other hand.

Scruff and Sit: An Alternate Technique.
1. Grasp and hold firmly a large amount of the loose skin (the scruff) behind the cat's neck.
2. With your other hand, hold the cat's body in a sitting position.

Minimal Restraint. Some cats are actually more easily managed with minimal restraint and gentle handling, and will become more difficult to handle with the above techniques. Become familiar with your cat's personality so you can assess the most effective capture and restraint techniques in an emergency.

Carrying and Transporting Techniques

If you suspect a back injury, see Broken Back or Neck, page 57, for the proper transport technique. You may also need to refer to Restraint Techniques, page 28.

Carry the cat in a box or carrier if available. Follow the instructions below if you must carry the cat in your arms.

1. Cradle the cat in your arms.
2. Place your hand around the cat's front legs, with one or two fingers between her front paws.

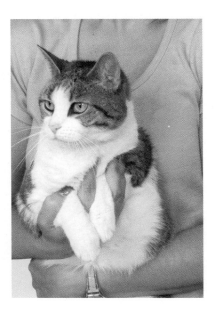

3. Support the hind legs with your other hand.
4. Keep the injured side against your body.

NOTE: Cats should always be transported in a box or carrier of some kind because they frighten easily and may jump out of your arms.

Be Prepared for Shock

Shock is the body's response to a change in blood flow and oxygen to the internal organs and tissues. It is always an emergency. It can result from a sudden loss of blood, a traumatic injury, heart failure, severe allergic reaction (anaphylactic shock), organ disease or an infection circulating through the body (septic shock). There are three stages of shock that may look very different:

- **Early shock** is when the body attempts to compensate for the decreased flow of fluids and oxygen to the tissues.
- **Middle shock** is when the body has difficulty compensating for the lack of blood flow and oxygen.

Is It an Emergency?

- **End stage shock** is when the body can no longer compensate for the lack of oxygen and blood flow to vital organs. This often leads to death.

See Shock, page 103, to learn how to respond.

Emergency Conditions
The following conditions are medical emergencies requiring immediate response:

- Birthing problems
- Bleeding that is prolonged or severe, such as spurting blood, or that you cannot stop by applying direct pressure
- Breathing difficulty
- Burns
- Cuts and gashes that expose internal organs or wounds with visible bone or severe tissue damage
- Drop in body temperature (hypothermia)

- Enlarged and/or painful abdomen
- Heat stroke (hyperthermia)
- Paralysis
- Poisoning
- Profuse diarrhea or vomiting
- Seizures, particularly first seizures; seizures lasting longer than 2 minutes; and repeating seizures (repeating one after the other)
- Severe depression (characterized by hiding, unresponsiveness or refusing to eat)
- Shock
- Snake bites
- Straining to urinate or defecate
- Trauma, such as being struck by a car, shot by a gun or falling from a significant height
- Unconsciousness

Call your veterinarian emergency hospital immediately if your cat is affected by any of these conditions.

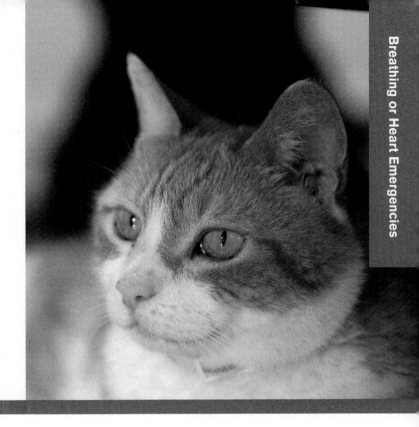

5

Respond to a Breathing or Heart Emergency

Breathing and heart problems are life-threatening emergencies in both man and animal. When seconds count, you won't have time to look up information in a book, so it's crucial to know how to respond before such an emergency occurs. Read this chapter carefully and watch the related segments on the DVD so you will know how to help your cat if he ever is in urgent need. This also is a good time to reflect on how well prepared you are to help your human loved ones in a similar emergency. Contact your local Red Cross chapter today and sign up for a CPR certification course.

Veterinary Emergency Numbers

Be prepared. Post your veterinarian's phone number, the local 24-hour emergency animal hospital phone number and the American Society for Prevention of Cruelty to Animals' Animal Poison Control Center's phone number (888-426-4435) near at least one phone in your house for easy reference. Make sure everyone in your household knows where to find the numbers.

You should also know where the closest 24-hour emergency animal hospital is so you won't get lost trying to get there when time is critical.

Cardiopulmonary Resuscitation

Cardiopulmonary resuscitation (CPR) is used to treat an animal that is not breathing and has no heartbeat or pulse. It consists of rescue breaths (also called mouth-to-nose or mouth-to-mouth breathing) and chest compressions. CPR is based on three basic principles, called the ABCs of CPR. Follow the A-B-C (Airway,

Breathing and Circulation) order when attempting CPR.

Airway

The airway is the breathing passage. To open the airway and check the throat and mouth for foreign objects, take the following steps:

1. Lay the animal down, on either side.
2. Gently tilt the head slightly back to extend the neck and head.
3. Pull the tongue between the front teeth.
4. Use your finger to check for and remove any foreign material or vomit from the mouth.

IMPORTANT: Do not place your fingers inside the mouth of a conscious animal—you may be bitten!

Breathing

After opening the airway, check to see if the cat is breathing. If the cat is not breathing, begin rescue breathing—

1. Cover and seal the cat's entire mouth and nose with your mouth and gently exhale until you see the chest rise.

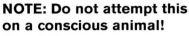

Cardiopulmonary Resuscitation

2. Give 4 or 5 breaths rapidly, then check to see if your pet is breathing without assistance. If he begins to breathe, but the breathing is shallow and irregular or if breathing does not begin, continue giving him rescue breaths at about a rate of 20–30 breaths per minute, pausing every 2-3 minutes to check for breathing and a pulse. Continue until you reach the veterinary hospital or for up to 20 minutes. Beyond 20 minutes, there is little chance of reviving your pet. (See Breathing Rate on Cat CPR Chart, page 36.)

NOTE: Do not attempt this on a conscious animal!

Circulation

Is there a heartbeat or a pulse? A cat's normal heart rate should be 160–220 beats per minute. If there is no heartbeat or pulse, perform chest compressions. (See Compression Position and Compression Rate on Cat CPR Chart, page 36.)

Hand Positioning. Here is how to best position your cat for CPR:

1. With the cat lying down on her right side, kneel with her chest facing you.
2. Place the palm of one hand over her ribs at the point

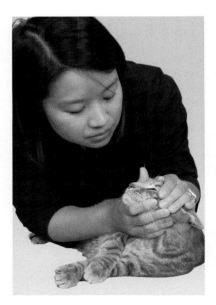

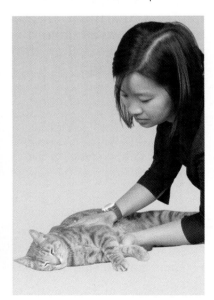

where her elbow touches the chest, just behind the front legs.
3. Place your other hand underneath her right side.
4. Compress the chest with both hands ½ to 1 inch or by 25–35 percent of her chest width.

Compression Rate. Compress the chest about 120–150 times per minute—or as fast as you can.

NOTE: Do not assume there is no heartbeat or pulse simply because an animal is not breathing. Do not start chest compressions before checking for a heartbeat. (If the animal is conscious and responds to you, then the heart is beating.)

Choking

Cats can choke on food or toys in an instant. But you can help your cat by knowing the signs of choking and following the steps below.

Signs and Symptoms.
• Anxiousness, cat acts frantic
• Cat stops breathing
• Gums may be blue or white
• Loud breathing sounds
• Pawing at the mouth
• Struggling or gasping to breathe

The Most Common Causes.
• Ill animal choking on her own vomit
• Object stuck in throat
• Tongue swelling due to an allergic reaction
• Trauma to neck or throat region

What You Can Do. Use caution to avoid being bitten, especially if working on a conscious or semi-conscious animal.

Open the mouth and carefully sweep the inside with your finger to try to feel and dislodge the object. Be careful not to push the object farther into the throat.

1. Pull the tongue forward, removing any object, vomit or foreign material present. (See Airway, page 32.)
2. Perform abdominal thrusts by lifting up the cat with the spine against your chest, place both of your hands around the animal's waist, or if she is conscious or struggling then hold the cat up by the scruff on the back of

her neck with one hand and use the other hand to perform an abdominal thrust.

- If using two hands for abdominal thrusts, close your hands together to make a fist and place the fist just behind the last rib. **(Step 2)**
- If using one hand to perform the abdominal thrust, place one fist behind the last rib while the other hand holds the cat up by the scruff on the back of her neck.
- Compress the abdomen by pushing up with your fist 5 times quickly and rapidly.

3. Carefully sweep her mouth with your finger to dislodge the object, if it has not already come out on its own.
4. If this is unsuccessful, suspend the cat by the hips with the head hanging down. **(Step 4)**
5. Next, check the animal's mouth again using a finger sweep and remove the object if possible.
6. If you cannot dislodge the object, give 5 sharp blows with the palm of your hand to the cat's back between the shoulder blades. **(Step 6)**

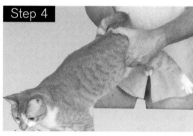
Step 4

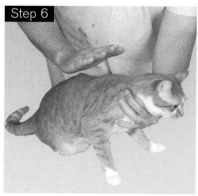
Step 6

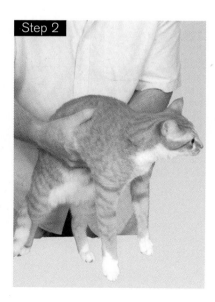
Step 2

7. Carefully sweep the cat's mouth with your finger to dislodge the object if it has not already come out on its own.
8. If the cat becomes unconscious, give 5 rescue breaths (see Breathing, page 32) and give 5 quick abdominal thrusts, then check the mouth again.
9. Once the object is dislodged, stop abdominal thrusts, check the cat's ABCs and begin CPR if needed. (See CPR, page 32.)
10. Take the cat to a veterinary hospital at once.

CAT CPR CHART

Breaths-to-Compressions Ratio	• 1 breath, then 5 compressions with 1 rescuer • 1 breath, then 3 compressions with 2 rescuers
Breathing Position	• Cover and seal cat's mouth and nose with your mouth, and gently exhale until you see the chest rise.
Breathing Rate	• Give about 4–5 breaths rapidly, then check to see if the cat is breathing on his own. • Give about 20–30 breaths per minute.
Compression Position	• With cat's chest facing you, place one hand over and the other hand under his ribs, just behind the front legs. • Squeeze your hands together. • Compress the chest about ½ to 1 inch (about 25–30 percent of his chest width) each time.
Compression Rate	• Perform 120–150 chest compressions per minute—or as fast as you can.
How Long Should You Perform CPR?	• Perform cycles of rescue breaths and chest compressions (CPR), then check for breathing and a pulse every 2–3 minutes. • If no pulse, continue CPR until the animal has a strong heartbeat and pulse, until you reach the veterinary hospital or until 20 minutes have passed and your efforts have not been successful.

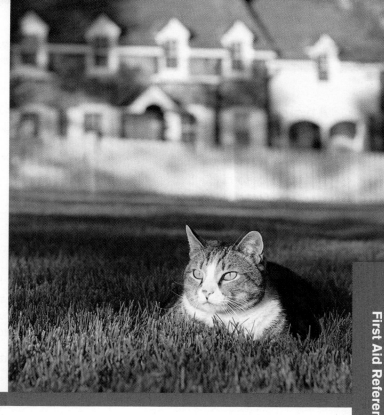

6

First Aid Reference Guide

If you turned to this section of the book because you are worried about your sick or injured cat, remain calm. Look for your pet's condition or symptoms; the topics are arranged alphabetically. Many subject areas will refer you to other topics, where you will find even more information you need to help your cat. You'll also find out if you need to take him to a veterinarian.

Abrasions

Abrasions—scrapes to the skin's top layers—can be shallow and heal easily or large and more serious. Your cat may lick or scratch the area, which may appear red or ooze blood.

What You Can Do.

1. Wash your hands and put on nonlatex, disposable gloves.
2. Apply a sterile, water-soluble (not petroleum-based) lubricant (see Pet First Aid Kit, page 16) so hair does not contaminate the wound while you shave the area.
3. Clip hair around the area gently with grooming clippers.
4. Flush the wound with warm water or saline solution (add 1 teaspoon of salt to 1 quart of warm water to make solution) to remove the skin lubricant.
5. Then wash the wound with water or saline solution to remove any remaining dirt or debris. If necessary, wet a gauze sponge with sterile saline solution to clean any remaining debris.

Take your cat to the veterinarian if the abrasion is larger than a quarter, seems painful, is red, does not begin to heal after 2–3 days, oozes a yellow or foul-smelling discharge or if you are unsure of its depth or severity.

Allergies and Allergic Reactions

Insect Bites

Although rare, cats can get spider bites and bee stings during the warm-weather months. Insects often sting or bite the soft, less hairy areas of your pet, such as the nose and feet. These sometimes cause allergic reactions.

Signs and Symptoms.

- Collapse (see Collapse, page 62)
- Difficulty breathing
- Pain, itching, licking at the site
- Redness, discoloration or hives (bumps in the skin) around the site, sometimes spreading to other body parts
- Red bumps on the abdomen, vomiting or diarrhea and swelling at the sting site, which may spread and include the face (especially around the eyes) and neck

NOTE: A severe allergic reaction can lead to anaphylactic shock. This could occur immediately or progressively over several hours. (See Shock, page 103.)

What You Can Do.

1. If your cat's face and neck are swollen, check her airway, breathing and circulation (ABCs). (See Airway, Breathing and Circulation pages 32–33.) If your cat cannot breathe, begin rescue breathing. (See Cardio-pulmonary Resuscitation [CPR], page 32.) If your cat's breathing is noisy or labored, take him to a veterinarian immediately.
2. Check for signs of shock. (See Shock, page 103.)
3. Check if the stinger is still present; it's usually black and very small. Do not attempt to pick it out, as this may release more of the toxin. Instead, scrape it off with a firm object, such as your fingernail or a credit card.
4. Apply a cool compress or ice pack wrapped in a towel to help control swelling.
5. Transport your cat to a veterinary hospital. (See How to Approach, Capture and Restrain a Cat, page 25.)
6. It may be appropriate to give your cat the over-the-counter antihistamine chlorpheniramine (Chlor-Trimeton®) **if your veterinarian has given approval.** Many over-the-counter products contain chlorpheniramine along with other cold or allergy medications (i.e., acetaminophen or pseudoephedrine). **It is extremely important to ensure that the product contains ONLY chlorpheniramine.**

Chlorpheniramine (Chlor-Trimeton®) Dosing. In general, the dose is 2 mg twice a day. **Give oral medication only if your cat is conscious, able to breathe and not vomiting!**

Skin Allergies

Allergies are one of the most common causes of skin conditions in cats.

Signs and Symptoms.

Itchiness; swelling; red skin; or red bumps, with or without a white center—*pustules* or *papules*, respectively—most commonly on the lower abdomen (belly)

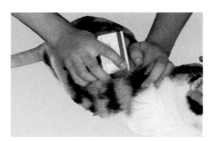

The Most Common Causes.
Flea bites, food, flea and tick products, grass, mold, pollen and other plants, grooming products and household cleaning products

What You Can Do.
1. Wash your cat thoroughly using a very mild soap or baby shampoo.
2. Apply a compress, such as a cool, wet washcloth, to the affected area.
3. Administer chlorpheniramine (Chlor-Trimeton®) if approved by your veterinarian.
4. Talk to your veterinarian about potential causes and treatment (i.e., flea treatment [see Parasitic Disease, page 88]). A secondary infection may develop, requiring oral antibiotics.

Anal Sac Swelling/ Infection/Abscess

If you notice your cat frequently licking at or scooting his hind quarters around the house, it might be because he's trying to express an impacted anal gland that's making him uncomfortable. Cats usually express these glands upon defecating. An impacted anal gland is not only painful, but it can become infected and abscessed.

Signs and Symptoms.
Anorexia, fever, lethargy, redness, pressure, pain, licking at and scooting the area, possibly discharge/pus on one side of the anus

What You Can Do. Take your cat to the veterinarian. If the gland is impacted, a veterinarian can express it. If it's infected or abscessed, the veterinarian will sedate your cat to lance and flush the swelling, then give oral antibiotics.

If your cat has an abscess that has not ruptured, take your cat to a veterinarian as soon as possible for abscess care. If the abscess has ruptured, clean the area as described under Abrasions, page 38, and take her to a veterinarian.

Prevention. Your veterinarian can check anal glands during checkups.

Balance, Loss of (Vestibular Disease)

Vestibular disease causes a cat to lose her balance. It occurs in cats of all ages and isn't always life threatening—even though it mimics a stroke. However, it is serious and needs immediate attention. Many cats with a less serious case compensate well and overcome it.

The Most Common Causes.
Brain disease, foreign object in the ear, inner ear infection, parasitic disease, a problem with the balance center in the brain (called idiopathic peripheral vestibular disease)

Signs and Symptoms.
Change in behavior, circling in one direction, drooling, eyes appearing to move rapidly from side to side or up and down, falling to one side, head tilting to one side, vomiting

What You Can Do.
1. Any animal with these symptoms should be examined by a veterinarian as soon as possible.
2. Look inside your cat's ears. If they are red, swollen or contain a lot of debris, he may have an ear infection. Take him to a veterinarian for treatment. Prolonged, untreated ear infections can lead to hearing loss or brain infections.

If the veterinarian diagnoses peripheral vestibular disease, it is crucial to keep your cat out of danger and away from stair-

cases, balconies and open windows. And don't allow him free reign outdoors. It is not known what causes idiopathic peripheral vestibular disease, but it tends to occur in the warmer months and is more common in older cats. The good news is that peripheral vestibular disease generally clears up on its own, in about 2–6 weeks. However, your cat must be examined by a veterinarian to rule out more serious brain diseases, including central vestibular disease.

Birthing Emergencies (Dystocia)
In a perfect world, every cat would have a home. Unfortunately, we don't live in that world. Spaying or neutering your cat is crucial to control pet overpopulation (and cat homelessness) and also has positive health and behavioral benefits. (See Spaying and Neutering, page 4.) But sometimes the unexpected happens. You may take in a stray or otherwise acquire a pregnant cat. If you suspect pregnancy, take the cat to your veterinarian for advice and treatment. Once you know she's pregnant, prepare in advance by providing a whelping box, bedding and a heat

First Aid Reference Guide

source. If you are faced with an unexpected birth, use the following information as a guide.

In cats, normal pregnancies last 62–64 days. About a day before giving birth, the cat's body temperature decreases to less than 100° F, she may have a decreased appetite and her nesting behavior (gathering materials for a bed) may get very intense.

Labor and Delivery
Stage one—the cervix dilates. The cat generally appears nervous or anxious and may pace, pant and lie down and get up a lot; this may last for 12–24 hours. Contractions will not be visible.

Stage two—forceful visible uterine contractions occur. She actively strains to expel each kitten. These contractions look as if she is trying to defecate while lying on her side, and she probably will pant. Stage two labor usually lasts from 3–6 hours, but it may last up to 10–12 hours or more if she is disturbed or is having a large litter. If the contractions are weak, a kitten could be born every 3–4 hours, but if contractions are strong and

forceful the kittens could be born about 30 minutes apart. The first kitten should be born within 1–2 hours after stage two labor begins.

Stage three—the placenta should come out with each kitten or shortly afterward. The whole process should last between 12 and 36 hours.

Normal Position of Kittens. Slightly more than half of kittens are born head first and the rest are born rear-end first. Both presentations are normal.

After Birth. The mother should clean off each kitten after it is born and sever the umbilical cord with her teeth. Usually, she will eat the placenta. The mother will have a red, brown or dark-green vaginal discharge (*lochia*), which may persist up to 3 weeks, but should become less profuse after the first few days. Take her to a veterinarian if this discharge appears bright red, contains pus or has a foul odor, as these are signs of infection.

Birthing Problems
The Most Common Causes.
- Deformed or dead fetus
- The mother's pelvis is too small, the kitten is too large or

the mother had a prior pelvic injury, such as a fracture
- Weak uterine contractions or twisted uterus

Signs and Symptoms.
- More than 2 days past the cat's due date or past a temperature drop (if known) or a dark vaginal discharge with a foul odor
- Active labor for more than 4 hours with no kitten
- More than 30 minutes of active continuous straining between kittens with no kitten produced (active straining is an obvious contraction with the cat trying to push)
- Kitten at the vulva, but mother unable to push it out within 20 minutes
- Mother looking weak, sick and depressed
- Mother biting or whining at vulva area
- Bloody discharge before birth

It is a good idea to check on your cat, but do not be overly attentive. If the cat is in active labor for 4 or more hours with no kitten, or she has any of the above signs, call a veterinarian *immediately* for an assessment, and be prepared to get her to a veterinary hospital. At the veterinary hospital, the attending doctor may

attempt to treat her with medication to increase the force of contractions. Otherwise, a cesarean section may be performed.

NOTE: Most cats will stop labor if they are disturbed.

What You Can Do. If the kitten is visible but the mother cannot push any longer—

1. Put on nonlatex, disposable gloves.
2. Gently grasp the kitten with a clean towel.
3. When the mother bears down (during an active contraction) help pull the kitten gently out of the vulva toward you in a slightly downward direction. **Do not pull the kitten when the mother is not pushing.** You can easily dislocate or fracture bones if the fetus is pulled too vigorously.

If the mother is not cleaning up the kitten—

1. Allow the mother to try to clean the kitten. If she doesn't, remove the kitten from the sac and clean the mouth, nose (to remove any fluid) and eyes with a clean cloth.
2. Rub gently (but vigorously) to stimulate breathing.

First Aid Reference Guide

3. Dry the kitten with a cloth. Cut the umbilical cord, but only after the kitten is breathing and its gums are pink.

To cut the cord properly—

1. Tie a piece of fishing line, dental floss or heavy string snugly around the cord about 1 inch from the body.
2. Make a second tie about a ½ inch from the first. (Do not pull on the cord as this can cause a hernia.)
3. Cut between the two ties.

If the kitten is not breathing—

1. Wipe kitten with a towel. Clear the face, nose, eyes and mouth.
2. Hold the kitten firmly in your hand with the head pointing down.
3. Clean away fluid from the nose and mouth. (You can suction gently with a baby dosing syringe or bulb syringe.)
4. If the newborn is still not breathing, perform rescue breathing. (See CPR, page 32.)
5. Repeat vigorous rubbing with a towel, holding the kitten on a slight downward slant to drain any fluids. Continue to perform rescue breathing as needed. (See CPR, page 32.) Do not shake or jostle the newborn.

If you suspect a problem, call your veterinarian immediately!

Bite Wounds

It's scary to see your cat engaged in a catfight and it can be extremely dangerous. But never try to break up a catfight yourself—you could be injured.

Bite wounds can look minor but can be deep and serious, so if your cat is bitten by another animal, take him to a veterinarian as soon as possible to prevent the wound from becoming infected. **This is especially true if your cat was bitten and shaken by a dog, which can cause significant internal injuries. Take him to a veterinarian immediately.**

Signs and Symptoms. Small wound in skin, most likely two puncture marks; bleeding; bruising

If a wound is not immediately apparent, the injured cat may develop an infection or abscess 1 or 2 days after being bitten.

Signs of bite wound infection include: fever, usually above 103° F; lethargy; loss of appetite; and pain when affected area is touched.

An **abscess** is a soft swelling around the wound. If unruptured, the top of the swelling may be red or blue, painful and look taut. If ruptured, pus will be visible, often accompanied by a foul odor.

What You Can Do.
1. If the wound is bleeding excessively, control the bleeding. (See Bleeding, this page.)
2. Check the cat's ABCs; perform CPR as needed. (See CPR, page 32.)
3. Check for shock. (See Shock, page 103.)
4. Administer basic wound care. (See Abrasions, page 38.)

If you witness the bite, find out the rabies vaccination status of the attacking cat or animal if possible. Recheck the rabies vaccination status of the bitten cat. If your pet was bitten by a wild animal and the wild animal is dead, call your veterinarian or Animal Control officer so it can be sent to a laboratory for a rabies examination.

If you suspect a snakebite, see Venomous Bites and Stings—Snakes, Scorpions and Toads, page 110.

NOTE: To dispose of a dead, wild animal, wear nonlatex, disposable gloves and place the animal in a plastic bag, then seal the bag. Do not attempt to capture a live wild animal.

Bleeding
There are two types of serious bleeding: arterial bleeding, characterized by rhythmically spurting blood, is more rapid and profuse and therefore more difficult to stop; and venous bleeding, which is slower and less profuse, much easier to stop and less dangerous, unless a large vein is involved.

(For nosebleeds, see Nosebleeds, page 87. For bleeding ear flaps, see Ear Problems, page 67.)

What You Can Do.
1. Wearing nonlatex, disposable gloves, hold a piece of gauze, washcloth or other clean material over the bleeding site and apply direct pressure. **(Step 1)** If the material becomes soaked through, do not remove it but apply another

cloth over it. Do this repeat-edly if necessary. Direct pressure is the safest way to stop bleeding until you can reach a veterinary hospital.

2. If bleeding has not stopped and blood is spurting, in addition to direct pressure over the wound, hold the area just *above* the wound with your hand in an effort to close off the blood vessels. If blood is flowing heavily but not spurting, hold the area just *below* the bleeding site to close off the blood vessels.

3. If this fails to stop the bleeding, apply a pressure bandage.
   - Wrap gauze or other soft material around the wound just tight enough to stop the bleeding. Do not make it too tight. **(Step 3A)**
   - Secure with tape or cohesive wrap. **(Step 3B)**
   - If you wrapped a limb, check repeatedly for swelling of the toes or toes that become cold; these signs indicate your bandage

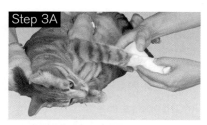
Step 3A

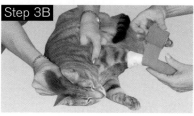
Step 3B

is too tight, in which case you will need to loosen it.

4. If the limb does not appear to be broken, elevate the limb above the heart, while continuing to apply direct pressure.

5. If none of the above techniques work, apply hand pressure to pressure points (see below).

6. Take your cat to a veterinarian immediately.

Pressure Point Technique
To help control bleeding, you can use the pressure point technique. Apply firm, even pressure to the appropriate pressure point:

- **Bleeding on the front limbs.** Press three fingers up and into the armpit on the side with the bleeding limb.

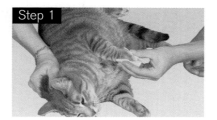
Step 1

- **Bleeding on the back limbs.** Press three fingers on the area of the inner thigh where the leg meets the body wall on the side with the bleeding limb.
- **Bleeding of the head.** Press three fingers at the base of the lower jaw (the angle just below the ear) on the same side and below where the bleeding is occurring.
- **Bleeding of the neck.** Press three fingers in the soft groove next to the windpipe (which feels round and hard) just below the wound on the side of the neck where the bleeding is occurring. Be sure not to apply pressure to the windpipe itself.

When using pressure points to control bleeding, you must release pressure slightly, for a few seconds, at least every 10 minutes. This helps prevent permanent damage.

IMPORTANT: Avoid using the neck pressure point on any animal suspected of having a head injury, unless you feel the animal's life is in immediate danger. Be sure you do not restrict breathing.

Tourniquet Technique
Use only on the limbs—never place a tourniquet around the neck!

1. Wrap a strip of cloth or gauze (about 2 inches wide) twice around the limb above the bleeding area. **DO NOT MAKE A KNOT.**
2. Tighten the gauze or cloth by wrapping each end around a rigid object, such as a stick.
3. Turn the stick slowly and just enough to stop the blood flow. Write the time on a piece of tape on the tourniquet.
4. Loosen the tie for several seconds at least every 10 minutes to help avoid permanent tissue damage.
5. Be aware that the interrupted blood supply may cause your cat to lose the limb.
6. Take your cat to a veterinarian immediately.

NOTE: Pressure points and tourniquets should be used only as a last resort, in a life-or-death situation. (For example, the animal has lost enough blood to lose consciousness.) Persistent decreased blood flow to the area may cause severe damage.

First Aid Reference Guide

Blood Calcium, Low, Eclampsia (Following Birth)

Eclampsia, or low-blood calcium, may occur in female cats during late pregnancy and up to 2–4 weeks after giving birth. It's much less common in cats than in dogs, but it's worth taking note of, as it can be life threatening; it can cause the lactating cat to be unable to meet the increasing demands of blood calcium or move calcium into her milk supply without depleting it in her own blood. Low blood calcium can also be caused by acute kidney failure, poisons, pancreatitis or other diseases.

Calcium is needed for muscle activity, so muscle tremors and seizures can occur when the blood calcium level drops sharply.

Signs and Symptoms. Muscle tremors, which may involve the whole body; seizures; fever; restlessness; nervousness; stiff gait or inability to walk

What You Can Do.
1. Take your pet to a veterinary hospital immediately.

2. Kittens should stop nursing and be given a supplemental formula. Ask your veterinarian for instructions on how to do this.

Prevention. Feed a pregnant cat kitten food 2–3 weeks before delivery and continue for 4 weeks after delivery. Have your cat spayed.

Blood in Urine

Red-colored urine signals the presence of blood and is probably due to urinary tract disease. It could also indicate a bladder stone, tumor or even poisoning. So it's important to get your cat to a veterinarian as soon as possible to determine the cause. If your cat is straining to urinate and you are unsure if he is adequately passing urine, take him to a veterinarian immediately. (See Urinary Blockage, page 108.)

The Most Common Causes. Bladder inflammation, stones or infection; kidney infection; poisoning (rat poison); trauma; tumor; uterine infection in a female cat

What You Can Do.
1. Watch carefully to be sure your pet is able to pass or produce urine.

2. Check for other signs, such as vomiting, lack of appetite or lethargy.
3. In the case of a nonspayed female, look at her vulva to see if there is a discharge; if the discharge contains pus and smells foul, she may have a uterine infection known as a *pyometra*. (See Vaginal Discharge and Uterine Infection, page 109.)
4. Take your cat to a veterinarian. If possible, bring a new, clean urine specimen from the animal.

NOTE: To collect a cat's urine specimen, replace your usual cat litter with a nonabsorbent material (such as fish-tank gravel). After the cat urinates, pour the urine out of the litter box and into a clean container. It is best to obtain the specimen the same day you go to the veterinarian, but if this is not possible, you can place the specimen in the refrigerator overnight.

Prevention. Spay your female cat to prevent uterine infections. If your cat is being treated for a urinary tract infection, administering your pet's antibiotics as prescribed can help prevent future infections. Also, adhere to any special diet or other medication your veterinarian prescribes.

Blood in Stool
Signs and Symptoms. Bright red blood in or on top of stool or—more serious—melena, a black, tarry stool

The Most Common Causes. Colitis; straining while defecating; stomach ulcer or tumor causing bleeding in the upper intestines

What You Can Do. Call the veterinarian immediately whenever you observe blood in your cat's stool.

Blood Sugar Emergencies
Blood sugar emergencies can be life threatening and are often caused by diabetes. They can occur abruptly if the blood sugar level is too high (*hyperglycemia*) or too low (*hypoglycemia*). It's important to monitor your pet's glucose level (usually in urine) if she is diabetic. Most diabetic cats require insulin injections once or twice daily, although some may be regulated through oral medications or diet alone.

First Aid Reference Guide

Hyperglycemia

Hyperglycemia is when the blood sugar level is too high. One of the most common causes of hyperglycemia is *diabetes mellitus*, which is the abnormal metabolism of insulin. If a diabetic cat's blood sugar is too high and he develops another health problem, he can go into a diabetic ketoacidotic state. This is a life-threatening emergency.

Signs and Symptoms of Hyperglycemia. Increased appetite, increased thirst, increased urination, weight loss

If your cat has diabetes and progresses to a diabetic ketoacidosis state, other signs can occur, including—

- Change in behavior.
- Dehydration. (See Dehydration, page 64.)
- Increased breathing rate.
- Loss of appetite.
- Shock and death, if untreated.
- Sweet smell to breath (ketones).
- Weakness.
- Vomiting.

Causes of Hyperglycemia Due to Diabetes Mellitus.

Inadequate insulin regulation, undiagnosed diabetes mellitus, incorrect insulin dose, increased insulin demand, insulin not properly administered

Causes of Hyperglycemia Not Due to Diabetes Mellitus.

Glandular or endocrine disease; organ disease or stress; less commonly, if a cat gorges on a bulk food source

What You Can Do.

1. Check the cat's ABCs; perform CPR as needed. (See CPR, page 32.)
2. Check for shock. (See Shock, page 103.)
3. Take your cat to a veterinary hospital as soon as possible. Be sure to take her insulin and syringe with you.

Hypoglycemia

Hypoglycemia occurs when the blood sugar level is too low. The most common cause is insulin overdose in a diabetic cat.

Signs and Symptoms. Coma or unconsciousness; disorientation; seizures; shaking; weakness; wobbly, drunken looking

Causes of Hypoglycemia Due to Diabetes Mellitus or Receiving Insulin.

- Not eating after receiving an insulin injection (always feed your pet prior to giving him insulin)
- Overdose of insulin, which can be caused by the wrong insulin syringe being used, a change in the type of insulin being used or improper administration
- Reduced need for insulin
- Vomiting up a meal after receiving an insulin injection

Causes Of Hypoglycemia Not Due to Diabetes Mellitus or Receiving Insulin.

- Severe infection/sepsis
- Liver disease
- Loss of appetite—mostly in young kittens
- Poor nutrition in very young animals
- Tumor that secretes insulin

What You Can Do.

1. Check the cat's ABCs; perform CPR as needed. (See CPR, page 32.)
2. Rub corn syrup on the gums, but do not force it into the mouth. Do this even if your pet is comatose. An oral glucose paste is sold at pharmacies; if you know your pet is diabetic or has a history of low blood sugar, keep this product in your first aid kit.
3. If you do not have the glucose paste or corn syrup, rub sugar water on the gums.
4. Take the animal to a veterinary hospital immediately.

Bone, Dislocated (Out of Joint)/Subluxation

The two most common joints to become luxated (completely dislocated) are the hip and elbow. Congenital disease and trauma can cause an elbow to become luxated. Trauma can also cause a luxated hip joint. In any case, your cat must be seen by a veterinarian immediately.

Signs and Symptoms.
Hip

- Animal feels pain when you feel or touch the area
- Dislocated hind leg is shorter or longer than the other
- Foot on dislocated leg does not reach the ground when the animal stands

Elbow

- Animal feels pain when you feel or touch the area
- Elbow is bent
- Foot does not reach the ground
- Lower leg is pointed away from or toward the body

First Aid Reference Guide

What You Can Do.

1. Check the cat's ABCs; perform CPR as needed. (See CPR, page 32.)
2. Check for shock. (See Shock, page 103.)
3. Transport your cat to a veterinary hospital as soon as possible. The sooner you get her to the hospital, the greater the chance the bone can be placed back in the joint without surgery.

Bone, Muscle and Joint Injuries

Sprains and Strains

A sprain is an injury involving a ligament (the tissue that connects bones to bones or bones to muscles). A strain is an injury to a muscle.

Signs and Symptoms.

- Limping (not placing the limb down at all or placing less weight on it)
- Pain when the area is touched
- Swelling

What You Can Do.

1. Apply either a cool compress (ice pack or chemical cold pack) or a warm compress to the injured area three or four times daily, for 5–15 minutes each time. Alternate warm and cold, using warm for one application, then cold for the next. Place a towel between the compresses and the skin.
2. Restrict exercise. Keep the animal in a small, closed, confined area.
3. If there is no improvement in 24 hours, or if the injury worsens, seek veterinary attention. An x-ray will need to be taken to make sure there are no fractures or torn ligaments.

IMPORTANT: Never give aspirin or any other over-the-counter pain relievers to your pet unless prescribed by your veterinarian. These drugs can be very toxic, even fatal! One Tylenol® tablet can kill a cat.

Fractures

Fractures are breaks in the bone. They may occur singularly, in one part of the bone, or there may be multiple breaks in the bone or multiple bones involved. Fractures can have smooth, clean surfaces or have splinters and fragments.

Fractures are assessed for severity based on—

- Location of the fracture.
- Whether a joint is involved.

- Whether it is a clean break (there may be chips or splinters present).
- Whether the fracture is straight or at an angle.
- Whether the fracture site is closed or open (with bone sticking through the skin).
- Whether the growth regions of the bone are affected, in the case of young animals.

Signs and Symptoms.
- Disfigurement (part of the limb seems to be abnormally positioned)
- Lameness (not placing full weight on a limb)
- Pain
- Piece of bone sticking through the skin
- Possible bruising (which can be difficult to see under the fur)
- Swelling

What You Can Do.
1. Keep your cat as quiet and calm as possible.
2. Check the cat's ABCs; perform CPR as needed. (See CPR, page 32.)
3. If a piece of bone is protruding from the fracture site—
   - Wash the area with water or saline solution (add one teaspoon of salt to a quart of warm water to make solution). (The animal may not allow this.)
   - Loosely place a dressing over the wound, extending several inches past the opening. Preferably use a sterile dressing, such as a nonstick pad or a gauze sponge, or use any clean piece of cloth.
   - Wrap the ends of the dressing with tape. Extend the tape several inches past the opening. Make sure you do not disturb the bones or wrap the dressing too tightly.
4. If you cannot transport your cat in a box, carrier or cage, or otherwise keep him completely still, you can try to splint the fracture (see below).

Splinting
Splints are placed to keep the fracture immobilized to prevent further damage, and can be used for fractures at or below the elbow and at or below the knee.

To correctly immobilize a fracture, the joints above and below the fracture site must be included in the splint.

1. After washing and dressing the area as discussed in Step 3 (above), splint the limb in the position you find it.

First Aid Reference Guide

2. Place a rigid structure along one or each side of the fractured limb. You can use sticks, tongue depressors or pens. **(Step 2)**
3. Place a strip of adhesive tape on each side of the foot, starting several inches above the wound and extending several inches past the end of the foot. These will act as stirrups, keeping the bandage in place.
4. Hold the splint in place with tape placed at multiple sites surrounding the splint and limb, or bandage the splint in place with roll gauze, starting at the toes and extending up. **(Step 4)**
5. Do not disturb the bones—try to hold both sides of the fracture steady and don't wrap too tightly. Pull the ends of the sticky tape over the end of the gauze roll bandage as far as it will go, with the sticky part twisted to face and adhere to the bandage.
6. Place an elastic or cling roll bandage over the roll gauze starting at the toes. **(Step 6)**

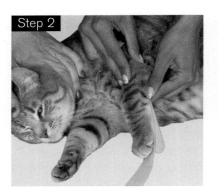

Step 2

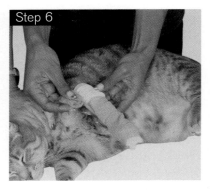

Step 6

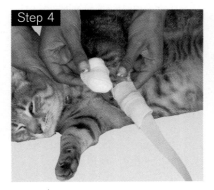

Step 4

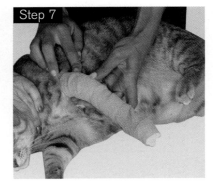

Step 7

7. Make sure the tape or bandage is not too tight that it cuts off circulation. Check by placing two fingers between the tape or bandage and the limb. **(Step 7)**
8. If no rigid material is available, a splint can be made by wrapping the limb with layers of a cloth, such as a towel, and taping the cloth in place. Only splint a fracture if it is below the elbow or knee— you can not immobilize a fracture on the upper limbs.

If a hip or shoulder is broken, transport your cat to a veterinary hospital immediately in a small carrier or box.

NOTE: Splinting a limb incorrectly can cause more damage. If you are unsure about splinting a limb or if your cat struggles too much, it is better to transport the pet in a box or carrier, or in a way that prevents your cat from moving around, on the way to the veterinary hospital.

Breathing Problems

When your cat has a breathing problem, it is very important to first make sure that she's not choking. If she is, see Choking, page 34. If she's not choking but is having trouble breathing, get her to the nearest veterinary hospital immediately.

Signs and Symptoms.
- Abdomen moves when breathing
- Increased breathing rate and effort
- Loud, noisy breathing
- Open-mouth breathing
- Pale or blue gums (mucous membranes; see Know What's Normal, page 22)

The Most Common Causes.
- Asthma
- Cancer
- Electrical shock
- Fluid in the space around lungs (pleural effusion)
- Heart disease/congestive heart failure (see Heart Disease and Cardiac Emergencies, page 80)
- Inhaled objects or vomit
- Lung infections such as pneumonia
- Trauma (i.e., hit by a car)
- Upper airway disease
- Upper respiratory infection

Feline Asthma
Feline asthma can be caused by allergies, but often an underlying cause is not found.

Signs and Symptoms.
- Increased breathing rate
- Increased breathing effort, especially when exhaling

- Open-mouth breathing
- Cyanosis (blue color to mucous membranes)
- Staying in one place
- Wheezing (a musical sound heard when the cat breathes)
- Grunting when exhaling
- Coughing (may sound as if the cat is trying to cough or gag up a hairball)

NOTE: The cat may seem completely normal between episodes.

What You Can Do.
1. Check the cat's ABCs; perform CPR as needed. (See CPR, page 32.)
2. **Take the cat to a veterinary hospital immediately.**
3. Limit activity by confining the cat in a box or carrier during transport. Manual restraint can make a cat very uncomfortable.

Prevention. While there is no foolproof prevention method, if the asthma is associated with allergies, there are many things you can do to decrease the risk of acute attacks, such as—

- Don't allow anyone to smoke in your cat's environment.
- Decrease or eliminate the use of aerosols in the house, including hair sprays, deodorants and perfumes.
- Use only mild carpet detergents and avoid carpet powders.
- Avoid pine cleaners.
- Clean litter boxes with mild soap and water only.
- Use dust-free litters.
- Keep the cat indoors.

NOTE: Cats kept indoors enjoy longer, healthier lives than cats allowed to roam outside.

Pleural Effusion
Pleural effusion results from an accumulation of fluid in the space around the lungs.

Signs and Symptoms. Lethargy; short, shallow breaths; not wanting to walk around; open-mouth breathing

The Most Common Causes.
Heart disease, feline infectious peritonitis, cancer, infection

What You Can Do. Take your cat to a veterinarian immediately. The veterinarian will remove the fluid from the space between your cat's lungs and chest wall. This will make him more comfortable. This fluid will be analyzed to obtain a diagnosis and treatment plan. Your cat also may need additional tests such as chest x-rays, chest ultrasound and a cardiology consult.

Upper Airway Obstruction
The Most Common Causes.
- Nasopharyngeal polyp or mass
- Airway tumor
- Airway foreign body
- Upper respiratory tract infection

What You Can Do.
1. Check the cat's ABCs; perform CPR as needed. (See CPR, page 32.)
2. Allow the animal to assume the most comfortable position in which to breathe.
3. Transport your pet to the nearest veterinary hospital. Use a carrier or box if possible.

Broken Back or Neck
A broken back or neck in a cat is a very serious injury. Your cat may be in extreme pain so it's very important to carefully muzzle her to protect anyone who's trying to help. (See How to Approach, Capture and Restrain a Cat, page 25.)

Signs and Symptoms.
- Dribbling urine or feces
- Divot (area that appears lower) on the cat's back
- Inability to move head, front or hind legs or both

- Open anus
- Pain
- Stiff, extended front legs

What You Can Do.
1. Check the cat's ABCs; perform CPR as needed. (See CPR, page 32.)
2. Try to slide a board under your cat, keeping him as still as possible:
   - Place a board up on its side along the back of your cat.
   - It is best if the head, chest and legs can be held to prevent movement.
   - Then lower the board and, at the same time, slide the cat onto it, keeping the body and head as still as possible.
   - Secure your cat to the board by placing tape or torn strips of cloth over him and around the board.
   - Transport him to a veterinary hospital immediately.

Bruises
Bruises may not be obvious, but if your cat is favoring one side or another, she could have one.

Signs and Symptoms. Hematoma (blood-filled swelling) or seroma (serum-filled swelling) under the skin; red to purple marks on the skin; swelling

The Most Common Causes.
Bleeding disorder, cancer, mild blunt trauma (i.e., bumping into something)

What You Can Do.
1. Discuss the appearance of the bruised area with your veterinarian.
2. Apply cool compresses to the area four or five times a day for 15 minutes until the swelling goes down (may take several days for a seroma or hematoma).
3. Bruising can also indicate a clotting problem. If you have any question about the cause of the bruising or if there are multiple bruises, take your cat to a veterinarian.

Burns
(Major and Minor)
Cats are notorious for jumping onto hot stoves and catching their tails on fire, as well as seeking out warm car engines in the cold weather. Both can lead to burns.

Burns are classified by severity depending on their depth and the percentage of surface area affected. Superficial burns that are extensive can be as dangerous as deep burns affecting a small area. Severe burns can lead to shock and place your cat at risk for significant infection and potential death.

First Degree—Burns Involving Only the Superficial Layers of Skin
Superficial burns generally heal well with veterinary care.

Signs and Symptoms. Singed fur, reddening of the skin, swelling, tenderness or pain

Second Degree—Burns Involving Deeper Layers of the Skin
Deep burns usually heal well, but there may be some skin scarring.

Signs and Symptoms.
Blisters, loss of fur, redness, swelling, tenderness

Third Degree—Burns Involving All Layers of the Skin, as Well as Blood Vessels, and the Tissues and Cells of the Skin Are Destroyed
Deep burns involving blood vessels often heal with a lot of scarring. Intensive care and even surgery may be required.

Signs and Symptoms. Loss of skin, skin is not sensitive to touch, swelling under the skin, area looks charred (black and leathery) or whitish

What You Can Do.

1. Check for the signs of shock in the case of deep or extensive burns. (See Shock, page 103.)
2. Cool water should be applied as soon as possible. This decreases pain and may decrease the penetration of heat further into the tissues. If the burn involves only one body part, you can immerse your cat in a cool bath.
3. If more than one body part is affected, do not immerse your pet. Instead, run cool water directly over the areas or place cool compresses on the areas. Immersing a cat with extensive burns may cool the skin too quickly and cause shock.
4. Place a sterile nonstick pad or clean moist cloth over the burned area to keep it clean.
5. Take your cat to a veterinary hospital immediately.

NOTE: Do not place any ointments, butter or petroleum jelly on burns.

Car Accidents

For their protection and safety, cats should be indoor companions. However, even indoor cats sometimes escape to the dangerous outside world where they are struck by cars. So be diligent in keeping your indoor cat indoors. Also, whenever you transport her in the car, always use a cat carrier. Here is some information that will help you know how to respond if your cat is ever hurt in a car accident. Be sure to also take her to a veterinarian immediately to check for internal injuries.

The Most Common Causes.

- Escaping from inside the house or being allowed to roam free and running into the path of a vehicle
- Jumping out of a car window
- Being struck by a vehicle as it's backing up

What You Can Do.

1. If you witness the event, try to make a mental note of exactly where on her body your cat was hit, and whether she was simply struck or was driven over. Also note whether or not she was thrown. Often, even in very serious cases, a cat will get up and attempt to walk away. This does not necessarily mean she was not severely injured; this is an instinctive response in

which an injured animal tries to escape danger.

2. Approach the scene cautiously. Alert oncoming traffic. If traffic has not stopped, try to take your cat safely to the side of the road before examining her. It's preferable to always place a muzzle on your injured cat. If you do not have time to assess how best to carry the cat, follow the steps in the section entitled Carrying and Transporting Techniques, page 29. Take care to not worsen any obvious fracture or limb displacement.

3. If your cat cannot move or appears to have a spinal injury, place her on a flat board for transport. (See Broken Back or Neck, page 57.) If you cannot find a board, use a blanket or shirt (slide your cat onto it and have one or two people hold it on each side as stiffly as possible). If the cat cannot move, she may have a broken back or severe internal injuries, and she may be in shock.

4. Assess and note the position of the cat and the presence of blood, urine or feces (the veterinarian will need this information when you get to the hospital).

5. Does your cat have an open airway? Is she breathing? Or is her breathing labored? Is there a heartbeat or pulse? If not, see CPR, page 32.

6. If alert and standing, observe whether your cat is limping or favoring one side. Look for blood, open wounds, bruising or limbs hanging in abnormal positions.

7. If your cat is bleeding, see Bleeding, page 45.

8. Check for shock. (See Shock, page 103.)

Any cat that has been hit by a car should be taken directly to a veterinary hospital. Many internal injuries caused by the trauma may not show up for 12–72 hours after the incident. These can include slow leakage of blood from internal organs, rupture of the urinary bladder or other internal organs and air or blood leaking into the chest cavity. Because the cat's body is initially attempting to compensate for the trauma, early shock may be difficult to identify.

Prevention.
- ALWAYS be sure to look around and under your car before backing up.
- KEEP your cat as an indoor pet and make sure she wears a break-away (to prevent choking), reflective collar.

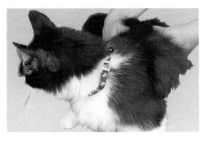

Choking
See "Choking" in Chapter 5: Respond to a Breathing or Heart Emergency, page 34.

Close Encounters (Skunk, Porcupine)
Cats that are allowed to roam outside may encounter certain wildlife—such as skunks or porcupines—that can lead to very unpleasant consequences.

Skunk
If your cat encounters a skunk, you will never forget the smell. Although being sprayed isn't life threatening to your cat, the skunk spray can irritate his eyes as well as yours. The smell is difficult to remove and gets tougher the longer it stays on your pet without treatment. So act quickly!

What You Can Do. You will need to wash your cat in tomato juice or an over-the-counter cat shampoo/degreaser (you can

even combine them). It may take several washings.

Porcupine
Porcupines, most commonly found throughout the Pacific Northwest and most of North America, are vegetarian rodents known for their unique coat, consisting of about 30,000 quills. Contrary to popular belief, porcupines do not shoot or eject their quills. When they feel threatened, tiny muscles in the skin make the quills "stand up" in defense. A swipe of their tails leaves a bunch of needle-like quills in whatever the tail happens to touch.

What You Can Do. If your cat has only a few quills and you are certain none are embedded in the mouth or throat, you can try to remove them with a pair of pliers. However, this will be a painful experience for your cat, so have someone help you restrain him.

1. Cover your cat's eyes so he doesn't see the pliers approaching and speak to him in soft, soothing tones.
2. Firmly grab the quill with the pliers close to the skin. Your cat might jerk backward, separating himself from the quill.

3. If there are numerous or deeply embedded quills, or if quills affect your cat's eyes, mouth or throat, take him to your veterinarian immediately where he will have the benefit of anesthesia and pain medications during the removal procedure.

Collapse

A cat that collapses is in serious trouble. She may be in shock or be beginning to have a seizure. Regardless of the cause, assess your cat to see if she needs CPR and take her to a veterinarian immediately.

Signs and Symptoms.

Extreme (profound) weakness, sudden falling over, loss of consciousness

The Most Common Causes.

- Abnormal heart rhythm
- Anemia
- Occasionally a primary orthopedic or neurological problem leading to not wanting or being able to get up
- Diabetes (See "Diabetes Mellitus" in Blood Sugar Emergencies, page 50.)
- Difficulty breathing
- Heart disease (See Heart Disease and Cardiac Emergencies, page 80.)
- Kidney or liver failure

- Severe blood loss—external or internal into the abdominal cavity (i.e., from a ruptured tumor of the abdomen), into the gastrointestinal tract, into the chest cavity or into the area around the kidneys
- Seizures (See Seizures, page 101.)
- Shock (See Shock, page 103.)

What You Can You Do.

1. Check the cat's ABCs; perform CPR as needed. (See CPR, page 32.)
2. Check for shock. (See Shock, page 103.)
3. Take your cat to a veterinary hospital immediately.

Constipation

Even your furry family member can become irregular from time to time. Most of the time, it's nothing to worry about. But in some instances, a cat may have colitis, which is an acute or chronic inflammation of the membrane lining the colon. It causes straining while defecating and mimics constipation. So if the constipation goes on for more than 24 hours, take your cat to the veterinarian. Cats are also prone to certain health conditions that make it much more difficult for him to defecate.

Signs and Symptoms.
- Crying while straining to defecate in the litter box
- Vomiting and decreased appetite
- Small, very hard stool

The Most Common Causes.
- Change in daily routine
- Colitis
- Dehydration
- Dirty litter box
- Dysfunction of the neuro-muscular system of the intestines
- Eating something inappropriate
- Excessive grooming or eating hair
- Not eating
- Tumors

What You Can Do. If your cat is still passing stool but it appears very firm and he is otherwise healthy (normal eating and drinking), try to add ¼ teaspoon of fiber (such as canned pumpkin or bran) to his diet. If adding fiber to the diet does not work, he is straining to defecate or he appears ill, take him to a veterinarian.

IMPORTANT: Never use commercial enemas made for humans! These may be toxic and deadly to cats!

Cuts and Tears (Major and Minor Lacerations)

Lacerations are wounds that cut through the skin to the deeper underlying layers. They may be deep enough to involve underlying veins, arteries, nerves, ligaments, muscles, tendons or even bone. It is crucial to assess your cat's condition and to see the extent of the laceration so you can treat it the right way. If it's minor, you can treat it at home; if it's major and bleeding heavily, take your cat to a veterinarian.

Signs and Symptoms.
- Bleeding (There may be a great deal of bleeding if an artery was cut.)
- Licking or limping
- Open wound (Underlying structures such as ligaments or muscle may be visible.)

The Most Common Causes.
Accidental injury, trauma, animal abuse, animal fights

What You Can Do. First aid depends on the extent of damage, the degree of bleeding and the cause of the laceration. If there is profuse bleeding, do not attempt to scrub the wound, as you will encourage more bleeding. You should flush the wound with large amounts of water or

First Aid Reference Guide

sterile saline solution, pouring it over the wound but not touching the wound. If the bleeding is not excessive, clean the wound (see Abrasions, page 38). If the cause is a bite wound, see Bite Wounds, page 44.

1. Check the cat's ABCs; perform CPR as needed. (See CPR, page 32.)
2. Check for shock. (See Shock, page 103.)
3. Stop the bleeding. (See Bleeding, page 45.)
4. Even if there is no bleeding, cover the area with a clean cloth until you get to a veterinarian.
5. Transport to a veterinary hospital, as many lacerations will require sutures/stitches.

Dehydration

Dehydration is the excessive loss of body fluids and can result from fever, vomiting and diarrhea; not eating or drinking; and increased urination, as well as too much heat exposure.

Signs and Symptoms.
- Change in urination habits (more or less)
- Excessive thirst and mouth dryness (i.e., dry, tacky gums)
- Loss of skin elasticity
- Sunken eyes

How to Determine Dehydration
Pull up on the skin at the back of your cat's neck; it should spring back to the normal position immediately (within 1 or 2 seconds). If it doesn't, she is dehydrated. Very old (geriatric) and very skinny cats are difficult to assess because skin loses some of its natural elasticity with age and malnourishment. It is also more difficult to assess dehydration in obese animals. In these circumstances, feel the gums; if they feel dry and sticky, your cat is probably dehydrated.

NOTE: If your cat is drooling, gums may feel moist even though she's actually dehydrated.

The Most Common Causes. Excessive heat exposure, illness—not eating or drinking, vomiting, diarrhea, fever

What You Can Do. A dehydrated cat must be taken to a veterinary hospital for treatment to determine why and how severely she is dehydrated. If she is vomiting or not eating/drinking, she will most likely need fluids either under the skin (subcutaneously) or intravenously. If you aren't sure whether or not your pet is dehydrated, the safest option is to take your pet to the veterinarian for an examination.

Dental Disease, Tooth Damage and Mouth Sores

It can be difficult to tell if a cat has tooth damage or dental disease. Paying attention to the signs of dental disease and treating your cat's mouth problems now could prevent him from having bigger health problems later on, because mouth infections can travel through the bloodstream and cause organ damage.

Signs and Symptoms.
- Bad breath
- Cracked or broken tooth
- Drooling or difficulty chewing
- Plaque buildup that looks brown or yellow
- Recessed, reddened gums or mouth sores
- Refusing to eat

The Most Common Causes.
Lack of regular dental care, accidents, injury

What You Can Do. Have your
cat's teeth checked during his regular checkups to determine if they need to be cleaned with an ultrasonic cleaner (similar to the one your dentist uses). Brush your cat's teeth regularly if he allows you to. Starting at an

early age will allow him to get used to you brushing his teeth.

Diarrhea

Diarrhea is an increase in the amount, fluidity or frequency of bowel movements. If it lasts for more than 24 hours, call your veterinarian.

The Most Common Causes.
There are many causes of sudden diarrhea, ranging from your cat having eaten something disagreeable to the first signs of severe illness. A sudden change in diet can lead to stomach upset for your pet. A short list of possible causes includes—

- Chronic inflammatory disease (when the walls of the intestines become irritated and nutrients cannot be absorbed).
- Disease of an organ or organ failure, such as liver or kidney disease or inflammation of the pancreas (*pancreatitis*).
- Infectious disease (bacterial, viral and fungal infections).
- Parasitic infection (most common in kittens).
- Tumors in the stomach or intestines; cancer in any organ.
- Glandular disease (especially common in cats with over-active thyroid glands).
- Stress.

First Aid Reference Guide

- Dietary problems (most common), including eating something improper, such as food off the street or human food; a change in regular diet; or intolerance to previously eaten food.
- Toxin or drug ingestion. (See Poisoning, page 95.)

What You Can Do.

1. If the diarrhea continues for more than 24 hours; if your cat is very young (under 1 year), elderly (over 10 years) or otherwise sick; or if vomiting is associated with diarrhea, she should be checked by a veterinarian as soon as possible.
2. If the diarrhea contains blood—either fresh (red stool) or digested (black stool)—have your cat examined by a veterinarian.
3. Check vital signs such as temperature (see How to Take Your Cat's Temperature, page 24), mucous membrane color (see Observe Your Cat's Mucous Membrane Color, pages 24–25) or capillary refill time (see Capillary Refill Time, page 25). Also be sure to check for dehydration (see Dehydration, page 64). If any of these are abnormal, have your cat examined by a veterinarian.

4. Take away any possible culprit, such as a new food or a new toy, whose use coincides with the onset of diarrhea.
5. Switch to a high-fiber, low-fat or bland diet (see Bland Diet, below). If the diarrhea subsides after 2–3 days on the bland diet, slowly mix in your pet's regular food and wean back to a normal diet over the course of a week. If attempts to wean to a normal diet don't work and diarrhea resumes, have your cat examined by a veterinarian.
6. As long as there is no vomiting, provide as much water as your cat desires. **Do not withhold water from a cat that has only diarrhea (no vomiting) as this will quickly cause dehydration. For animals that are vomiting, see Vomiting, page 112.**

Bland Diet.

- Mix boiled chicken with skin, fat and bones removed, or boiled chopped or ground meat with fat drained off, with cooked white rice using a 1-part-meat to 3-parts-rice ratio. Alternatively, your cat may eat only the chicken without the rice.
- Use a special bland or high-fiber (canned or dry)

food purchased from your veterinarian.

NOTE: A bland diet should be used as a temporary measure only to control diarrhea or rest the digestive system after vomiting. It does not contain sufficient nutrients as a permanent diet.

Drowning

Always keep an eye on your cat when near any body of water.

The Most Common Causes.
- Animal abuse
- Disasters, such as floods
- Falling through thin ice or falling into water from which they cannot escape
- Cat left unattended during a tub bath

What You Can Do.
1. For an unconscious cat, lift your cat up by the hind legs (you can suspend him) to allow water to come out the nose or mouth.
2. Lay your cat down, on either side, with the head slightly lowered.
3. Check the cat's ABCs; perform CPR as needed. (See CPR, page 32.)
4. Place a blanket (thermal, if possible) around your cat.

5. Transport to a veterinary hospital immediately.

Even if you revive your cat, an examination by a veterinarian is still necessary because fluid buildup in the lungs, as well as the effects of hypothermia, may result. (See Hypothermia, page 83.)

Ear Problems (Infections, Injuries)

Ear problems are quite common in cats. Most of the time, the problems are harmless and you can treat them at home. But if it's a severe infection, it could affect your cat's hearing, so it's best to get her seen by a veterinarian.

Bleeding, Ear Flap
What You Can Do.
- Apply direct pressure to the bleeding site with a cloth or piece of gauze for 5 minutes.
- If the bleeding does not subside, take your cat to the veterinarian.

Ear Infections
Ear infections can range in severity from superficial infections to deep infections that can cause hearing loss and balance problems.

First Aid Reference Guide

Signs and Symptoms.
- Foul odor coming from the ear
- Head shaking or head tilt
- Scratching at ear
- Material in the ear (may be black, brown, white or look like pus)
- Pain when touching the ear
- Red swollen ear, with possible blood

The Most Common Causes.
- Ear mites—a common parasite that is very contagious, especially in overcrowded conditions
- Allergies—flea, food or inhalant (pollen, grass, etc.)
- Infections from bacteria, yeast or parasites

What You Can Do. Have your cat examined by a veterinarian to determine the cause of the ear infection and prescribe the appropriate medication.

Prevention.
- Keep any cat diagnosed with ear mites away from other animals.
- Keep your cat's ears clean.
  - Use gauze sponges to clean ears.
  - Never place cotton swabs into the ear canal. You may push debris further into the ear.

- Never attempt to go deeper into an ear than you can see.
- Ask your veterinarian to show you how to clean the ears safely.

Swollen Ear Flap (Aural Hematoma)
An aural hematoma is a collection of blood between the layers of the cat's ear.

The Most Common Causes.
Chronic head shaking from an ear infection, trauma, bleeding disorder

Signs and Symptoms.
Swollen, soft and squeezable ear flap and infection. (See Ear Infections, page 67.)

What You Can Do. Take your cat to a veterinarian. This condition generally requires the ear flap to be drained surgically.

Prevention.
- Have ear infections treated as soon as they occur.
- If your cat is prone to ear infections, then once or twice weekly clean your cat's ears with a veterinary product that breaks up ear wax. (Ask your veterinarian to recommend the best product for your pet.)

Electric Shock (Electric Cord Bites)

Although not very common, electric shock or electrocution injuries occur when inquisitive cats or—more commonly— kittens bite electric cords.

Signs and Symptoms. Some signs occur immediately; others may not be obvious for hours or even days.

- Collapse on the floor near an electrical cord
- Difficulty breathing and coughing due to a buildup of fluid in the lungs
- Drooling
- Foul odor from the mouth
- Ulcers inside the mouth affecting the tongue, roof, cheek and gums
- Possibly part of the tongue missing
- Loss of appetite
- Shock (See Shock, page 103.)

What You Can Do.

1. Turn off the power and unplug the cord. If you cannot turn off the power at the source, turn off the power to the house.
2. Check the cat's ABCs; perform CPR as needed. (See CPR, page 32.)
3. Check for shock. (See Shock, page 103.)
4. Take your cat to a veterinary hospital immediately.

IMPORTANT: Do not attempt to free your cat from the cord if the power is on and the cord is still plugged in.

Prevention. None of these techniques are foolproof, but they may help.

- Use plastic sleeves or cord covers to prevent access to electric cords. These are available at hardware or computer stores.
- Place cords in inaccessible locations whenever possible.
- Unplug all electrical cords when not in use.
- Provide appropriate toys for chewing kittens.
- If you see your pet showing interest in a cord, rub the cord with a hot pepper sauce or other deterrents, such as Bitter Apple® (available at pet supply stores).

Eye Emergencies

If your cat's eyes are red, he should be examined by a veterinarian to make sure no sight-threatening conditions exist.

Acute Blindness

Acute blindness is most often detected when the cat starts bumping into things, is

First Aid Reference Guide

reluctant to go up or down stairs or is walking gingerly in the surrounding environment.

Signs and Symptoms.
- Bumping into furniture and walls
- Decreased appetite
- Dilated pupils (will look all black) that do not constrict with light
- Other neurological signs like seizures and abnormal behavior
- Reluctance to go up or down stairs or not wanting to walk around

The Most Common Causes.
- Primary eye problems
  - Chronic disease that appears more acute (i.e., progressive retinal atrophy)
  - Detached retinas, glaucoma, severe corneal ulcers or tumors
  - Infection or inflammation inside of the eye
- Primary neurological problems
  - Primary brain disease (infection, inflammation, tumor)
- Other problems
  - Low blood sugar

What You Can Do. Any cat with decreased or absent vision should be taken to a veterinar-

ian as soon as possible. In many cases, the primary cause needs to be found and treated to try to preserve vision. Always pay attention to how your pet is acting and if there is a difference in behavior when exposed to dark light versus bright light.

Conjunctivitis

Conjunctivitis is a swelling of the pink tissue lining the inside of the eyelids (*conjunctiva*). The conjunctiva can be seen by pulling down the lower eyelid and pulling up the upper eyelid.

Signs and Symptoms. Watery, mucus or pus discharge from the eye; eye that appears painful, itchy, red and/or swollen

The Most Common Causes.
- Infection (bacterial, viral or fungal)—especially common in young animals and can be contagious to other cats
- Defects in the eyelids (predisposed in some breeds)
- Chemical irritation or a foreign object in the eye
- Lack of tear production

What You Can Do. Have your cat examined by a veterinarian as soon as possible.

Eye Out of Socket (*Proptosis*)

Signs and Symptoms. One or both eyes bulging out of their sockets or other signs of trauma or pain

The Most Common Causes. These injuries are most often caused by trauma (i.e., hit by car, bite wounds). It takes a significant amount of force to cause proptosis to a cat's eye; therefore, head trauma is usually evident as well.

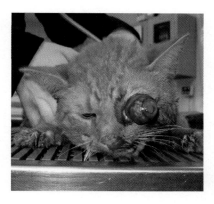

What You Can Do.

1. Administer sterile eye wash or sterile petroleum-based eye ointment (artificial tear preparation; available in pharmacies) to help keep the eye from drying out while transporting your cat to a veterinary hospital.
2. **Transport your cat as soon as possible to a veterinary hospital.** There may be significant head trauma that occurred with the proptosis. A veterinarian will decide whether it is feasible to try to put the eye back versus removing it. If the eye is put back, it is to try to save the eye—not the vision.
3. Place your cat in a box or carrier or carry your pet, if you must.
4. Keep your cat from pawing or scratching at the eye.

Foreign Objects in the Eye

Foreign objects are most commonly found on the *cornea* (the outer layer of the eye) or the conjunctiva.

Signs and Symptoms.

- Obvious foreign object
- Pawing at an eye
- Red or runny eyes, squinting or swelling

The Most Common Causes. The most common foreign objects in the eye are pieces of plant material, but there are many other objects that can get lodged in the eye. Normally, objects enter the eye either from flying debris or from brushing against a plant.

What You Can Do.

1. Gently wash the eye with large amounts of either tap water or sterile saline eye

wash. (See Administering Eye Medications, page 10.) Sterile saline eye wash is preferable; it is available at any pharmacy and should be a part of your first aid kit. (See Pet First Aid Kit, page 16.)

2. Inspect the eye with a good light source to ensure that the entire foreign object is gone.
3. Even if you are able to remove the foreign object, you should contact your veterinarian. Many foreign objects can cause a corneal ulcer or lead to infections. Your veterinarian may prescribe topical antibiotics.

If you are unable to remove the object with a stream of liquid, if it appears to be perforating the eyeball or if the eye looks very irritated, take your pet to a veterinary hospital immediately.

Glaucoma
Glaucoma is increased pressure inside the eye caused by a build-up of fluid.

Signs and Symptoms.
- There is an apparent change in vision.
- Cornea may be cloudy.
- Eye may appear enlarged or pupil may be dilated.

- Cat displays lack of appetite, lethargy, whining or crying, all of which are symptoms of pain (acute glaucoma may be very painful).
- Pupils may be unequal in size.
- Cat may have red or runny eyes.
- Cat may demonstrate sensitivity to light or squint.

The Most Common Causes.
- Infection or inflammation inside of the eye
- Tumor or cancer inside the eye
- Displaced eye lens
- Breed predisposition (Burmese, Siamese, Persian)

The diagnosis of glaucoma must be made by a veterinarian. It involves measuring the pressure inside the eye with an instrument called a tonometer.

What You Can Do. Acute glaucoma is a medical emergency; take your cat to a veterinary hospital immediately. Your cat will probably have to stay in the hospital to receive topical and intravenous medications to reduce the pressure in her eye in order to save her vision. Many animals eventually require surgery to correct glaucoma. Glaucoma is usually secondary to another disease in cats, so that disease process will need to be treated as well.

Ulcers, Corneal

Corneal ulcers are defects on the outer layer of the eye.

Signs and Symptoms.
- Cloudiness over the eye
- Discharge (watery, mucus or pus)
- May see the defect in the cornea
- Pain, redness, sensitivity to light or squinting

The Most Common Causes.
- Scratch, usually from another animal
- Foreign object
- Infection (bacterial, viral or fungal)
- Eyelashes that grow inward
- Decreased tear production
- Masses (tumors) on the eyelids

What You Can Do. Corneal ulcers are extremely serious. If left untreated, they can affect vision, rupture and cause the loss of the eye. Here is what to do.

1. Take your cat to a veterinary hospital immediately.
2. Prevent your cat from rubbing the eye. You may want to use a special device called an Elizabethan collar. (See Elizabethan Collars, page 12.) These are available from your veterinarian or pet supply store. It fastens around your cat's neck and extends around your cat's head like a cone. The purpose is to keep him from rubbing or scratching the eye.

Fading Kitten Syndrome

Fading kitten syndrome usually occurs in the first few weeks of life. The exact cause is not known and there probably are many factors involved. Unfortunately, it is associated with a high mortality rate.

Signs and Symptoms.
- Cannot keep temperature elevated even with a heat source
- Diarrhea
- Low blood sugar leading to wobbliness and decreased mentation
- Not active, gaining weight or nursing/eating

The Most Common Causes.
- Congenital abnormalities
- Inadequate nursing
- Infection—viral and/or bacterial
- Sick mother

What You Can Do.

1. Ensure that the mother is healthy, up to date on vaccinations and receives adequate nutrition.
2. Ensure that the kitten is getting enough nutrition/nursing adequately. Add kitten milk replacer through a bottle if necessary.
3. Weigh kitten daily to ensure she is gaining weight.
4. Make sure room temperature is correct. (Kittens cannot maintain body temperature for the first few weeks.)

Falling (High-Rise Syndrome)

High-rise syndrome most commonly occurs in urban settings due to the risk of falls from tall buildings. Cats that can fit through railings are especially at risk for this condition. Cats will often fall with legs in a downward position, with their neck and chin toward the ground.

Signs and Symptoms.

- Broken teeth
- Difficulty breathing—commonly due to air leaking from a damaged lung
- Fractures or dislocations of the limbs
- Jaw fractures
- Shock and internal injuries
- Split in the roof of the mouth

The Most Common Causes.

Animal abuse; falling or jumping from a window, terrace or other significant height

What You Can Do.
Cats that survive a fall often will attempt to run away afterward. This does not mean they are not seriously injured.

1. Survey the area for safety as you approach.
2. If the cat is not visible, check the entire area around the fall site, including bushes, brush and under cars.
3. Approach the cat cautiously. (See How to Approach, Capture and Restrain a Cat, page 25.)
4. Check the cat's ABCs; perform CPR as needed. (See CPR, page 32.) Take particular care when opening the mouth, because a jaw fracture may be present.
5. Control any bleeding. (See Bleeding, page 45.)
6. Check for shock. (See Shock, page 103.)
7. If emergency intervention is not needed on the spot, transport the cat to a

veterinary hospital
immediately.
8. Your transport technique
must take into account the
suspected injury. A box or
carrier is best. (See Carrying
and Transporting
Techniques, page 29.)

Prevention.
- Always keep screens on
open windows securely fas-
tened.
- Don't allow cats on terraces
or balconies that are not
screened.
- Don't leave windows open
wide enough for your pet to
squeeze through.

Fever
See How to Take Your Cat's
Temperature, page 24.

Fishhook
Injuries/Penetration
Cats are curious creatures. If a
cat smells a recently used fishhook, he may eat the hook to
get the fish remnants or he
might eat a fish that still has
the hook in its mouth. These
fishhooks usually are caught in
the cat's face and muzzle,
inside the mouth or on his paw.
It is also possible for a cat to
swallow a fishhook.

Signs and Symptoms.
- Fishhook protruding from
the skin; fishing line protruding from the mouth or anus
- Loss of appetite, painful
mouth or excessive drooling

The Most Common Causes.
- Accidental injury
- Playing with or sniffing fish-
ing equipment
- Swallowing a baited hook

What You Can Do. Your cat
should be taken to a veterinarian
for hook removal. If it is not possible to get him to a veterinarian
immediately, try the following:

1. Push the hook through the
exit wound until the barb is
visible.
2. Cut the barb off with a wire
cutter.
3. With the barb removed, pull
the hook out backwards, the
way it went in.
4. Treat like a wound. (See
Puncture Wounds and
Embedded Object, page 99.)
5. Even if you successfully
remove the hook, take your
cat to a veterinarian for
wound assessment and
possible antibiotic therapy.

If the hook is embedded
inside the mouth or if fishing
line is attached to a hook and

First Aid Reference Guide

swallowed, immediately transport your cat to a veterinary hospital where surgery may be performed. **Do not attempt to pull out the hook!**

Foreign Objects (Skin, Eye, Mouth, Nose, Throat, Swallowed)
Skin

Splinters and thorns are common foreign objects, as are sticks and glass. They can be found anywhere on cats.

Signs and Symptoms.
- Bleeding
- Licking at a paw
- Not placing any weight, or placing less weight, on a limb
- Obviously protruding thorn or other object
- Swelling at the site of the foreign object

The Most Common Causes.
- Accidental injury
- Running into a sharp object, such as a stick or fence
- Encounter with a porcupine (See Close Encounters, page 61.)

What You Can Do.
1. Sterilize a pair of tweezers and a needle, either by passing them through a flame or by dipping them in an alcohol solution.
2. Direct a good source of light to the area.
3. With the ends of the tweezers, take hold of and pull out the object. If it breaks, or if there are deep fragments, particularly of glass, do not attempt to remove them. Take your cat to a veterinary hospital for removal.
4. If the splinter is just below the surface of the skin, try to scrape the overlying skin with the needle and then grasp the object with the tweezers.
5. After removing the object, soak the affected area in a dilute solution of warm (not hot) water and Epsom salts for 15 minutes. Repeat this three or four times daily until the healing is complete.
6. If your cat had a foreign object stuck in her paw, do not use clay litter in the litter box until the wound heals over. (Cats sometimes react to changes in litter by refusing to use the litter box. If this occurs, talk to your veterinarian.)
7. If the wound is deep, if you cannot remove the entire object or if your cat does not put weight on the limb, take your cat to a veterinary hospital.

8. Also see Puncture Wounds and Embedded Object, page 99.
9. Discuss the injury with your veterinarian. Antibiotics may be required.

NOTE: Run your hands lightly over your cat's head, body, legs and feet every day to check for foreign bodies, injuries or parasites. Your cat will love the extra contact and affection!

Eye
See Eye Emergencies, page 69.

Mouth
While not as common as other injuries, cats can experience mouth injuries and objects can become stuck in the mouth or throat.

The Most Common Causes. Blades of grass that get stuck in the mouth or toys that injure the mouth

Signs and Symptoms. Drooling, not wanting to eat, pawing at the mouth

What You Can Do. Look inside your cat's mouth and check the roof of the mouth. Try to get the object out with your fingers, but if he seems distressed, call your veterinar-

ian. It may require sedation to remove the object.

Nose
Objects can become lodged in the nose.

The Most Common Causes. Blades of grass and grass awns

Signs and Symptoms. Nasal discharge, sneezing excessively

What You Can Do. Supervise your cat while outside.

Throat
See Choking, page 61.

Swallowed, Foreign Objects
Signs and Symptoms. Refusal to eat, vomiting

The Most Common Causes. Swallowing string, sewing needle with or without thread, toys (e.g., toy mice)

What You Can Do.
1. Call your veterinarian to discuss the object that was swallowed.
2. Bring your cat to the veterinarian if she is showing signs, such as vomiting, lack of appetite or lethargy. (See Vomiting, page 112.)

Frostbite
Sure, your cat has fur to help protect him from the elements,

but that doesn't mean he can't succumb to frostbite, which is actually the freezing of a body part or exposed skin and is a common occurrence in cases of acute hypothermia. (See Hypothermia, page 83.) The body parts most susceptible to frostbite include your cat's tail, tips of the ears and the pads of the feet. In the winter, if your cat goes outside, be sure to regularly check his feet for signs of frostbite.

Signs and Symptoms.
- Discoloration of the frozen area; skin that is pale or even blue in color initially, looking black and dead in later stages
- Lack of pain or sensation at the affected area, or a lot of pain, especially when the area starts to warm up

The Most Common Causes.
The causes of frostbite are the same as those for hypothermia. (See Hypothermia, page 83.)

What You Can Do.
1. Take your cat out of the cold.
2. Spray the affected area with warm water.
3. Lightly apply a warm compress to the area (ensure it is not hot enough to cause a burn). Do not rub or apply pressure to the area, as that could worsen the damage.
4. Transport your cat to the nearest veterinary hospital for care and to assess the affected area to see if there is permanent damage. If the tissue is dead, local amputation may be necessary.

Gunshot Wounds
Fortunately, gunshot wounds are not common injuries for our feline friends. If they do happen, however, assess your cat, perform CPR if needed and get him to a veterinarian immediately.

Signs and Symptoms.
- Lameness/fractures
- Profuse bleeding
- Signs of an entrance and/or exit wound
- Stumbling and falling to the ground

What You Can Do.
1. Your cat may attempt to run away; keep him as calm as possible.
2. Any part of the body may be affected, so it is important to examine him carefully and thoroughly. You may see a wound where the bullet pen-

etrated, or it may be difficult to find because it is covered by fur. Additionally, there may be a second wound where the bullet exited the body.

3. Check the cat's ABCs; perform CPR as needed. (See CPR, page 32.)
4. Try to stop the bleeding. Wearing nonlatex, disposable gloves, cover obvious wound sites with gauze, a nonstick dressing or a clean cloth and hold it in place. (See Bleeding, page 45.)
5. Check for shock. (See Shock, page 103.)
6. If the bullet has penetrated the chest and your cat is not breathing, perform rescue breathing (see CPR, page 32), and cover the chest wound with gauze or other clean material. These materials can be wrapped around the chest. Ensure that the wrap is not too tight to constrict chest movement.
7. With as little movement as possible, take your cat to a veterinary hospital immediately.

Head Entrapment

Cats can accidentally get their heads stuck in plastic or glass jars, leading to suffocation.

What You Can Do.

1. If it's a plastic jar, support the jar and head and use scissors or a screwdriver to punch holes in the jar so that the animal can get oxygen. You can also try to cut the jar in half.
2. If it's a glass jar, support the jar and head and gently tap the glass or use a hammer to break the glass so your cat can breathe.
3. Once there are holes or openings in the jar, use wire cutters, cardboard scissors or other scissors to cut off the rim of the jar. If possible, place a towel between the cat's neck and the rim.
4. Once the jar is off, if the cat is not breathing, check her ABCs and perform CPR as needed. (See CPR, page 32.)
5. Transport the cat to a veterinary hospital for evaluation. Suffocation, even for a small amount of time, can lead to fluid build-up in the lungs, requiring oxygen therapy.

Prevention. Keep all jars, particularly those that contain food, away from pets.

First Aid Reference Guide

Heart Disease and Cardiac Emergencies

Heart disease is quite common in cats. When his heart starts failing, a cat will experience congestive heart failure; the primary symptom is difficultly breathing. (See also Chapter 5: Respond to a Breathing or Heart Emergency, page 31.) Severe pain and paralysis can result if a blood clot forms in a cat's heart and lodges in his aorta, where it branches to the hind legs. This can occur in other parts of the body as well.

Signs and Symptoms.
- Fainting (uncommon in cats)
- Increased breathing rate or difficulty breathing
- Loss of appetite
- Lethargy/not wanting to walk around
- Open-mouth breathing
- Paralysis in the hind legs (less commonly, the front legs)
- Severe pain; the animal will cry out

The Most Common Causes.
- Abnormal heart rhythm
- Breed predisposition (such as the Himalayan)
- Cancer
- Cardiac birth defects
- Endocrine disorders such as hyperthyroidism

- Enlargement or dilation of the walls of the heart
- Improper nutrition
- Thickening of the heart muscle

What You Can Do.
1. Check the cat's ABCs; perform CPR as needed. (See CPR, page 32.)
2. Check for shock. (See Shock, page 103.)
3. In the case of cats that cry out and appear unable to move their hind legs, check for a pulse in the hind legs. (See Heart Rate and Pulse, page 23.) This pulse will be absent if there is a clot. Also, look at the color of the nails of the hind legs. Pink is normal and indicates blood is flowing to the area; white or blue nails indicate blood is not reaching that area. This foot may feel cooler to touch than the foot of the unaffected limbs.
4. Take your cat to a veterinary hospital immediately.

Prevention. Feed your pet high-quality food and take your pet for his annual veterinary checkups; it's the best way to find and follow heart murmurs or abnormalities.

Heat Stroke (Hyperthermia) and Heat Exhaustion

Heat stroke, or *hyperthermia*, occurs when a cat severely overheats—most often in the spring and summer months—when she has not yet acclimated to the hot weather. This condition is more common in outdoor cats and those left in a parked car. If the heat stroke isn't too advanced (with a body temperature of 104° F or above), you can help your cat recover.

NOTE: Make sure your pet has plenty of cool water and shade during hot weather.

Signs and Symptoms.
- Collapse
- Body temperature 104° F or above (See How to Take Your Cat's Temperature, page 24.)
- Bloody diarrhea or vomit
- Capillary refill time that is too quick (See Capillary Refill Time, page 25.)
- Depression, stupor (acting drunk), seizures or coma
- Excessive panting or difficulty breathing
- Increased heart rate (See Heart Rate and Pulse, page 23.)
- Increased respiratory rate (See Breathing Rate, page 23.)
- Mucous membrane color that is redder than normal (See Observe Your Cat's Mucous Membrane Color, pages 24–25.)
- Salivation

The Most Common Causes.
- A previous episode of heat stroke
- Cat left in a parked car
- Cat not acclimated to the warmer weather
- Lack of appropriate shelter for an animal outdoors
- Prolonged seizures
- Underlying disease state, such as upper airway, heart or lung disease

IMPORTANT: Never leave your pet in a parked car! Even with the windows cracked, your pet can quickly suffer heat stroke—and even die. Temperatures can exceed 120° F in parked cars!

What You Can Do.
1. Get your cat out of direct heat.
2. Check for shock. (See Shock, page 103.)

3. Take your cat's temperature. (See How to Take Your Cat's Temperature, page 24.)
4. Spray your cat with cool water. If using an outdoor hose, run the water to cool it off before spraying your pet. Spray her for a minute or two, then retake her temperature.
5. Place water-soaked towels on the cat's head, neck, feet, chest and abdomen.
6. Turn on a fan and point it in your cat's direction.
7. Immediately take your cat to the nearest veterinary hospital.

NOTE: The goal is to decrease the body temperature to about 103° F in the first 10–15 minutes. Once 103° F is reached, you must stop the cooling process because the body temperature will continue to decrease and can plummet dangerously low if you continue to cool the cat.

Even if you successfully cool your pet down to 103° F, you must take her to a veterinar-

ian as soon as possible because many consequences of hyperthermia won't show up for hours or even days. Some of these conditions can be fatal if not treated medically. Potential problems include—

- Abnormal heart rhythms.
- Blood clotting problems.
- Destruction of the digestive tract lining, leading to bloody vomiting and/or bloody diarrhea.
- Kidney failure.
- Neurological problems, including seizures and brain swelling.
- Respiratory arrest.

Hot Spots

While not common in cats, hot spots—inflamed areas of the skin—can result if your cat licks, bites or scratches an area too much. They can occur anywhere; but most of the time, hot spots form on the legs or hind end. They can have different degrees of severity depending on how long your cat has been aggravating the area. Typically, the lesions start as red or pink bald patches from your cat's biting and may end up bleeding and infected. So the earlier you catch them, the better for your cat.

Your cat may be creating a hot spot because he is bored. Combat boredom by providing him with safe toys he really enjoys, as well as exercise and lots of hugs and attention.

Signs and Symptoms.
Bleeding in the area, red or pink bald patches, discharge or foul odor from the area

The Most Common Causes.
- An area that may have originally been irritated by a sting or an external parasite, such as a flea, a foreign object, a scrape or an allergic condition
- Food allergies
- Psychological causes, such as boredom

What You Can Do.
1. Shave the area with grooming clippers.
2. Clean the area with warm water.
3. Look for the presence of any foreign objects, including insect stingers or fleas, and remove them.
4. Try putting an Elizabethan collar on the cat. (See Elizabethan Collars, page 12.) You can buy one from your veterinarian or a pet supply store. These collars fasten around your pet's neck and extend around the head like a cone. This keeps the cat from biting at most parts of the body and will prevent him from licking any topical treatment. Cats don't like wearing them, but they can help dramatically.
5. If topical treatments don't work, have your cat examined by a veterinarian.

Hypothermia (Dangerous Drop in Body Temperature)
Hypothermia is a drastic reduction of body temperature that happens when cats have been exposed to frigid temperatures for too long or if their fur gets wet in a cold, windy environment. When the body temperature drops, the heart rate and breathing slow down. The consequences of extreme hypothermia include

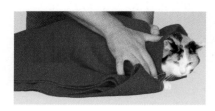

neurological problems (including coma), heart problems, kidney failure, slow or no breathing and frostbite. (See Frostbite, page 77.)

Signs and Symptoms.
• Body temperature below 95° F (See How to Take Your Cat's Temperature, page 24.)
• Decreased heart rate (See Heart Rate and Pulse, page 23.)
• Pale or blue mucous membranes (See Observe Your Cat's Mucous Membrane Color, pages 24–25.)
• Pupils that may be dilated (The black inner circle of the eye appears larger.)
• Shivering
• Stupor, unconsciousness or coma
• Weak pulse

The Most Common Causes.
• Falling into cold water or not being acclimated to the cold weather
• Inability to regulate body temperature (seen in very old and very young cats)
• Shock
• Stray or outdoor animal caught in the cold or a storm without shelter
• Underlying illness

What You Can Do.
1. Remove your cat from the cold.
2. Check the cat's ABCs; perform CPR as needed. (See CPR, page 32.)
3. Check for shock. (See Shock, page 103.)
4. Take a rectal temperature. (See How to Take Your Cat's Temperature, page 24.)
5. Wrap your cat in a blanket. (See Pet First Aid Kit, page 16.)
6. Place warm water bottles next to the cat, wrapping the bottles in towels to prevent burns.
7. Transport to a veterinary hospital immediately.

Insect Bites
See Allergies and Allergic Reactions, page 38; Parasitic Disease, page 88; and Venomous Bites and Stings, page 110.

Mammary Glands (Swollen or Red)
Mammary glands are located on the underbelly of a cat from the front armpits to the back legs and in females are used to feed kittens. When mammary glands are swollen, painful or red, the condition is called *mastitis* and is usually

due to a blocked milk duct. It may occur in female cats when they feed their kittens. Female cats can also develop mammary gland tumors.

Signs and Symptoms.
- Decreased appetite, fever, lethargy, vomiting
- Discharge from the gland (may look like milk with blood or pus in it)
- Swollen or red mammary gland that may or may not feel hot to the touch

The Most Common Causes.
- Dirty living conditions, infection or trauma from nursing kittens
- Pregnancy
- Tumor

What You Can Do.
1. Clean the nursing environment, including the whelping box, surrounding areas and anything that comes in contact with your cat.
2. Place warm compresses on the affected gland for 10–15 minutes every 3 or 4 hours.
3. Have your cat examined by a veterinarian who most likely will prescribe antibiotics if there is an infection.

Prevention. Keep nursing areas and living areas clean

and dry. Spay your cat at a young age to prevent pregnancy and the risk of mammary tumors.

Masses/Skin Swelling/Abscess, Lipoma or Tumor
Cats can get masses or swellings either in the skin or just under the skin (*subcutaneous*).

Signs and Symptoms.
- If in the skin, mass can look like a wart or pimple and be soft to firm.
- If under the skin, they can look like a swelling or ball-shaped mass.
- They may have a discharge.

The Most Common Causes.
- Abscess
- Fatty tumor under skin (Called a *lipoma*, it is benign and will feel soft. This is much less common in cats than in dogs.)
- Malignant mass in skin (*mast cell tumor*) or under skin

What You Can Do.
1. When petting your cat, feel through the fur coat to find small masses.
2. If one is found, write down where it is, its size and if it is firm or soft.

First Aid Reference Guide

3. Contact your veterinarian about *aspirating* the mass (sticking a needle into it to identify the cells and type of mass).
4. Monitor the size and tell your veterinarian if it is changing.
5. An abscess will be soft and the skin will most likely be red, hot and painful. If it has already ruptured, you might see pus or bloody discharge.
6. For a ruptured abscess, see Puncture Wounds and Embedded Object, page 99, for wound care and contact your veterinarian. The cat will most likely need antibiotics.
7. If not ruptured, contact your veterinarian.

Nails (Broken or Torn Toenails)

Your cat will most likely need regular nail trimming to prevent breaking or tearing. If your cat tears a nail, it will bleed and be painful, but it will grow back. Be sure to check the *dew claws* (the thumb toes higher on the foot) when trimming nails. Regularly clip only the sharp tips of your pet's nails using a clipper designed for cats. Your veterinarian can show you how.

Signs and Symptoms.
• Bleeding from the toe
• Licking
• Placing less weight on the leg with the broken toenail
• Shaking his paw

The Most Common Causes. Cutting a toenail too short during trimming, injury or not trimming toenails on a regular basis

What You Can Do. If the nail is bleeding, apply styptic powder to the area. This should be a part of your pet first aid kit (see Pet First Aid Kit, page 16). You can also try applying direct pressure to the nail with a piece of gauze or clean cloth for 5 minutes. If you do not have these items available, try the following:

1. Take a bar of soap and push it into the bleeding nail, or apply flour or cornstarch to the area with firm pressure for 5 minutes.
2. If you are not successful, wrap the paw. (See Pad Wounds, page 87.) After bandaging the paw, take your cat to a veterinary hospital.

Monitor the site for infection, as evidenced by swelling, pain, redness and reluctance to put weight on the paw. If any of these signs appear, take your cat to a veterinarian.

Nosebleeds

Usually nosebleeds happen only as a result of injury or blunt trauma. However, if there's a small amount of blood leaking from your cat's nostril without evidence of injury, this could be something more serious and she should be seen by a veterinarian as soon as possible.

Signs and Symptoms.

Bleeding from either or both nostrils

The Most Common Causes.

- Bleeding disorder
- Foreign object
- Infection, head trauma or injury
- Tumor

What You Can Do.

1. Apply an ice pack, wrapped in cloth, to the nose.
2. Place steady pressure on the bleeding nostril using a clean cloth or gauze.
3. Keep the cat as quiet and still as possible.
4. If the bleeding does not stop, is the result of anything but simple trauma (such as a thorn in the nose) or there is no obvious reason for the bleeding, immediately take the animal to a veterinarian for an examination. A small amount of blood from one nostril may be an early sign of a tumor or bleeding disorder.

Pad Wounds

The pads of your cat's feet contain many blood vessels that cause them to bleed heavily when injured.

Signs and Symptoms.

- Bleeding (may be heavy)
- Limping or not putting weight on the limb
- Wound or foreign object in pad

The Most Common Cause.

Stepping on a sharp object, such as a thorn or a piece of glass

What You Can Do.

1. Remove any obvious foreign object and try to stop the bleeding with direct pressure.
2. Wash the area with saline solution (to make solution, add 1 teaspoon of salt to 1 quart of warm water) or with warm, soapy water.
3. Dry the foot. Then apply an antibiotic ointment to prevent infection.
4. Bandage the foot by placing a strip of adhesive tape (see Pet First Aid Kit, page 16) on each side of the foot,

First Aid Reference Guide

starting several inches above the wound and extending several inches past the bottom of the foot. The tape on either side of the leg acts like stirrups to hold the bandage in place—the tape should go directly on the fur.

5. Place a nonstick pad or gauze sponge over the wound.
6. Wrap the paw with gauze roll (in the first aid kit), starting from the toes and ending just above the ankle or wrist.
7. Pull the ends of the sticky tape over the end of the gauze roll bandage as far as it will go, with the sticky part twisted to face and adhere to the bandage.
8. Place an elastic or cling roll bandage over the cotton, working from the toes to the ankle. Do not wrap tightly.
9. Make sure the bandage is not too tight; check for toe swelling and feel the limb just above the bandage for coolness, swelling or pain. If any of these are evident, loosen the bandage.
10. Take your cat to a veterinary hospital to get the wound assessed.

Parasitic Disease

Parasitic disease, including chiggers, fleas, intestinal worms, mites, ticks and toxoplasmosis, is not uncommon in cats. While some parasites don't cause too much concern, some of them can cause chronic disease. Read on about how you can detect and treat these pesky parasites in your feline friend.

Chiggers

These are common skin parasites found throughout the central and southern United States. They can bite and infect humans and cats and cause severe itching. They can be treated relatively easily.

Signs and Symptoms. Itching caused by small, reddish-orange mites about the size of a pinhead, resembling paprika, found on the legs, head and abdomen

The Most Common Causes. Walking through a chigger-infested area (Chiggers are found in grassy areas, mostly in the spring and fall.)

What You Can Do. Wash your cat with a mild shampoo. Contact your veterinarian about antihistamines or other treatments if symptoms are severe.

Fleas

Fleas are small, wingless insects with elongated back legs that allow them to jump onto a passing animal host. They feed on the blood of numerous animal species—including humans.

Signs and Symptoms.
- Intense scratching, sometimes accompanied by hair loss, redness and/or raised bumps on the skin
- Adult fleas or "flea dirt" (feces a female flea deposits when laying eggs) visible on cat

NOTE: Use a flea comb and water spray to search for evidence of fleas on your pet's head and hindquarters. Flea dirt will turn red when moistened because it is primarily digested blood.

The Most Common Causes.
Contact with a flea-infested animal or with flea eggs, larvae or pupae in your cat's indoor or outdoor environment.

What You Can Do. A flea infestation must address each one of the flea's four stages of development: eggs, larvae, pupae and adults. To be effective, you must treat both your cat and his environment.

- Talk to your veterinarian about the best way to treat your cat and other animals in the house.
- Thoroughly vacuum your home including behind and under furniture, drapes and your pet's bedding. Afterward, seal the vacuum bag in a plastic bag and discard it right away.
- Treat your home with a product that contains both an adulticide and an insect growth regulator that will kill adult fleas as well as stop the development of eggs and larvae.
- Clean and treat your automobile, garage, basement or any other place your cat frequents.
- Treat yard and kennel areas with an environmentally safe spray. Concentrate on areas where your cat spends most of his time outdoors, such as the patio, under the deck or porch and in and around the cat house. (Depending on the product used, you may need to repeat the yard treatment weekly or monthly.)
- Rake away and dispose of organic debris, such as leaves, weeds and grass clippings, to reduce the flea habitat.

First Aid Reference Guide

- Be persistent. It may take several weeks or even months to get rid of all of the fleas, in all life stages.
- Contract with a professional exterminator to treat severe infestations.

IMPORTANT: Read the label on all insecticides thoroughly and apply them as directed. Be especially careful if your household includes children, someone with asthma or pet fish or birds.

Prevention. The easiest and best way to control a flea infestation is to prevent one in the first place. There are a variety of flea control products you can use, including collars, sprays, dips, topical applications, shampoos and powders. There also are oral and injectable medications available. Ask your veterinarian which flea prevention and control method he or she recommends for your pet. Always talk to your veterinarian before using more than one product at a time.

IMPORTANT: Never use an insecticide intended for dogs on a cat.

Intestinal Worms (Roundworms, Hookworms, Whipworms)
Several different types of intestinal worms exist. These worms may be visible in the stool or they may be vomited up (more common in kittens). Roundworms look like pieces of spaghetti and hookworms can lead to significant blood loss if left untreated.

The Most Common Causes.
- Cats can pass the worms and eggs in their stool or vomit, and can acquire them easily by smelling or eating other animals' feces. It is best to assume that all the pets in a household are infected if one case of roundworms has been positively confirmed.
- Kittens get roundworms directly from their mother's milk when they start to suckle.

Signs and Symptoms.
- Anemia (pale gum color)
- Bloated abdomen
- Diarrhea, vomiting and weight loss
- Loss of appetite, or an animal that is very hungry but not gaining weight
- Poor-looking coat of hair

What You Can Do.

1. Take the animal to a veterinarian along with a stool sample. If you see worms in the vomit or stool, make sure the sample includes the worms.
2. Have your pet's stool checked for worms at her yearly physical examination or sooner if you suspect an infestation.

NOTE: It is very important to treat roundworm infections, as they may be transmitted to humans. Any pet that has been treated for worms should have a follow-up fecal examination to ensure the treatment was successful.

Prevention.

- Don't allow your cat to eat or sniff the feces of other animals.
- Don't introduce a new animal into your household without first having the animal checked and treated for worms.
- Have your pet's stool checked yearly by a veterinarian.

Mites and Mange

There are four different kinds of mange: sarcoptic, notoedric, demodectic and cheyletiella. Each one is caused by different species of mites—tiny, 8-legged creatures related to spiders.

Signs and Symptoms.

- Crusty ear tips
- Hair loss, sometimes spreading throughout the body
- Oozing sores or lesions
- Pin-point bite marks
- Secondary skin infection (in severe cases)
- Severe itching, especially on the elbows, ears, armpits, hocks, chest and abdomen (Mites prefer to live on skin areas with less hair.)
- Small, red pustules
- Yellow crust on the skin

Most Common Causes.

Sarcoptic mange, commonly known as scabies, is caused by the parasite *Sarcoptes scabiei*. These microscopic mites burrow into the skin of cats or kittens, where they lay eggs. Newly hatched mites continue tunneling under the skin. These mites can survive for several days off the host, so cats can become infected without ever coming into direct contact with an infected cat. This mite is also contagious to humans.

Notoedric mange is caused by *Notoedres cati*, a mite closely related to *Sarcoptes scabei*.

This causes mange similar to other mites and is more common in the Southwestern part of the United States.

Demodectic mange, also known as red mange or follicular mange, mostly plagues young cats. It is caused by the mite *Demodex gatoi*, which is transferred from the mother to offspring in the first few days of life. The first sign is hair loss, usually around the muzzle, eyes and other areas on the head. Sometimes this looks like a few circular crusty areas around the muzzle. In more severe cases, a cat could have generalized infestation all over the body.

Cheyletiella mange, also known as walking dandruff, affects kittens and cats. It is caused by a large, reddish mite that can be seen with a magnifying glass. This mange is identified by the dandruff-like dust that occurs over the cat's head, neck and back. It causes mild itching. Walking dandruff is highly contagious but short-lived. The mite that causes the mange dies soon after leaving the host.

What You Can Do. Mange can easily be mistaken for other skin conditions, making it impossible for pet owners to diagnose accurately. If your cat suffers from irritated, itchy skin, make an appointment with the veterinarian. Early diagnosis will give you a head start on a cure. Your veterinarian can prescribe topical, oral or injectable medications for mites.

In addition to treating the infestation itself, the veterinarian may prescribe antihistamines and steroids to help relieve your cat's itching. Antibiotic treatment also may be needed if a secondary infection has developed.

Ear Mites. The mite *Otodectes cynotis* takes up residence in an animal's ear canal. It is highly contagious and causes intense itching of the ears.

Signs and Symptoms.
- Scratching around the ears and/or frequent head shaking
- Fresh or dried blood visible inside the ear canal

NOTE: Dried blood resembles coffee grounds in the ear canal. If you notice this, your cat probably has ear mites.

Most Common Cause.
- Contact with another animal that has ear mites

What You Can Do.
- Check your cat's ears regularly for any discharge or redness.
- Talk to your veterinarian about how to clean your cat's ears safely at home

Tapeworms
Tapeworms are commonly spread when an animal bites an itch or eats fleas that harbor tapeworm larvae.

Signs and Symptoms.
- Round or flat small white worms that look like moving pieces of rice, which are segments of the tapeworm body, will be seen around the anus or in the stool.
- For other signs, see Intestinal Worms, page 90.

What You Can Do. Practice flea control and have your cat dewormed with medication administered by a veterinarian. Clean your animal's bedding thoroughly after starting treatment for tapeworms.

Ticks
Ticks are blood-sucking parasites responsible for the transmission of several diseases to dogs, cats and humans. They commonly jump on animals as they walk through tall grass or brush against leaves, bushes and trees. To get the most accurate information for your area, ask your veterinarian about diseases transmitted by ticks.

Signs and Symptoms of Tick Infestation.
- A tick may appear as a tiny, dark-colored insect or a fat, skin-colored bump; it is engorged with the cat's blood and has its head burrowed into the cat's skin.
- Ticks may be present anywhere on the body, but they are commonly found on the ears (or just inside them) and on the feet or legs.
- The area around the tick may be red and swollen.

What You Can Do.
- If you live in an area that has ticks, or after visiting such an area, check your pet thoroughly. Run your fingers through your pet's entire hair coat; check the paws by lifting each up and inspecting the pads; look between the toes and inside the ear.
- If you find a tick—
  1. Put on nonlatex, disposable gloves.
  2. Place a small amount of tick spray (available in

First Aid Reference Guide

pet stores or at your veterinary hospital) on a gauze sponge, cotton ball or paper towel and hold it over the tick. This will usually cause the tick to start to back out in 30–60 seconds.

3. When the tick starts to back out, grab the entire tick with a pair of tweezers.

4. Alcohol, mineral oil or petroleum jelly can be used in place of the tick spray, but they generally don't work as well. Don't use matches to singe the tick, as it may burn the animal's skin.

5. Flush the tick down the toilet or, if you are not sure what type of tick it is, you may want to save it in a secure container for identification by your veterinarian. (Different kinds of ticks carry a variety of diseases communicable to animals and humans.)

6. Apply a disinfectant, such as alcohol or an antibiotic ointment, to the site of the tick bite. A local skin reaction may occur around where the tick was attached.

Prevention. There are many products available for preventing ticks. Before using a tick product, check with your veterinarian to ensure it is safe for your cat's age.

Toxoplasmosis

Toxoplasmosis is caused by a microscopic parasite of cats. The primary risk associated with toxoplasmosis is that it can infect humans. If a pregnant woman becomes infected during the early months of pregnancy, it can cause serious fetal defects. People with suppressed immune systems are also at increased risk for this infection.

Humans become infected by ingesting infective eggs from the soil when gardening or by handling litter and not washing their hands before eating. However, the most common way humans become infected is not through contact with cats, but by eating undercooked infected meat. In the case of a pregnant woman, the cyst can cross the placenta to infect the fetus.

Signs and Symptoms in Cats. Eye infections, lung disease, seizures, vomiting or diarrhea, heart disease

The Most Common Causes.
- Eating undercooked meat (applies to animals and humans)
- Cats eating rodents or other infected prey
- Contact with egg-contaminated soil
- Playing in a sand box that an outdoor cat has used
- Passing from mother cat to offspring during pregnancy

What You Can Do. Take your cat to the veterinarian for diagnosis and treatment.

Prevention (For You and Your Cat).
1. Clean litter boxes daily. (It takes at least one day for eggs in feces to become infective.)
2. Have someone else change the litter box if you are pregnant or have a suppressed immune system.
3. Wear gloves and a surgical mask when cleaning the litter box.
4. Keep your cats indoors to decrease the risk of infection through hunting. Do not allow indoor cats to hunt mice or rats in the house.
5. Always wear gloves when gardening.
6. Discourage stray cats from using your backyard as a litter box. Cover sandboxes.
7. Don't eat raw or undercooked meat or feed it to your pets.
8. Wash hands frequently and thoroughly, especially after handling raw meat, cat litter or garden soil.

Poisoning
Because many plants can be poisonous to pets, ask your veterinarian which plants may be poisonous to cats or check the American Society for the Prevention of Cruelty to Animals' (ASPCA's) Web site (*www.aspca.org/toxicplants*) for a list of poisonous plants. Lillies are just one example of common houseplants that are very toxic to cats. So, before adding any plants to your home or garden, learn if it is harmful to your pet.

If you suspect that your cat has been exposed to any type of poison, call your veterinarian first. Then, if needed, contact the ASPCA's Animal Poison Control Center at 888-426-4435 for advice on what to do.

Signs and Symptoms.
Poisons can be eaten, inhaled or absorbed through the skin.

First Aid Reference Guide

tips

- [ ] You can now buy antifreeze that's much safer around animals and children who might accidentally ingest it. Look for antifreeze made with propylene glycol [not ethylene glycol, which is poisonous].

- [ ] Never give your pet any unprescribed medication without consulting a veterinarian. Over-the-counter medications for humans, such as ibuprofen and acetaminophen, are fatal to cats! (See Adverse Reactions from Human Medicines, page 13.)

- [ ] Always make sure the product you are using is appropriate for your animal, e.g., do not use flea products for dogs on cats—they will be toxic!

The signs of poisoning may occur immediately or within hours, or may take days to appear. They include—

- Bleeding from anus, mouth or any body cavity.
- Dilated pupils.
- Salivation (drooling or foaming at the mouth).
- Seizures or other abnormal mental state or behavior, such as hyper-excitability, trembling, depression, drowsiness or coma.
- Shock. (See Shock, page 103.)
- Swollen, red irritated skin or eyes.
- Ulcers in the mouth or burned lips, mouth or skin.
- Vomiting or diarrhea (with or without blood or particles of the ingested toxin).

The Most Common Causes.
- Accidental ingestion
- Animal abuse
- Eating food that may be toxic to a cat
- Eating garbage
- Improper medication given to a cat

Sources of Toxins
- Antifreeze (ethylene glycol)
- Drugs such as marijuana, cocaine, amphetamines and alcohol
- Heavy metals (i.e., zinc, lead)

- Household chemicals, including cleaning solutions, chlorine, lead-based paint and potpourri
- Household foods, including chocolate, onions and moldy cheese
- Inhaled toxins, such as carbon monoxide
- Many plants, both indoor and outdoor
- Non-prescription drugs, such as acetaminophen (Tylenol®) aspirin, ibuprofen (Advil®) or cold remedies
- Prescription medications, either an inappropriate dosage of medicine prescribed for the cat or medicine belonging to a human in the household and accidentally eaten by the cat
- Rat or mouse poison/bait or other pesticides, snail or slug bait, moth balls
- Topical products, such as flea powders, sprays, shampoos and dips—especially those containing pyrethrins, carbamates and/or organophosphates

What You Can Do.
1. Check the cat's ABCs; perform CPR as needed. (See CPR, page 32.)
2. Check the mucous membrane color. (See Observe Your Cat's Mucous Membrane Color, page 24.) Certain toxins cause specific changes in the color. For instance, cherry-red mucous membrane color occurs in cases of carbon monoxide poisoning.
3. Check the capillary refill time. (See Capillary Refill Time, page 25.)
4. Check the animal's mental state, looking for seizures, increased excitement, unsteadiness, depression or coma.
5. Call your veterinarian or veterinary emergency hospital. Your veterinarian may have you call the ASPCA's Animal Poison Control Center (888-426-4435) before coming to the hospital.

In either case, have the following information on hand, if possible:

- Exact name of the poison
- How much the animal ate or was exposed to
- How long ago exposure or ingestion occurred
- The animal's vital signs (temperature, heart rate, breathing rate, capillary refill time and mucous membrane color)
- Approximate weight of the animal

First Aid Reference Guide

At home, you will only be able, at best, to assist in ridding the pet's body of the toxin, depending on the type of poison. For specific types of poisoning, follow the information below.

Topical Poisons

1. Call your veterinarian or the ASPCA's Animal Poison Control Center for information about the specific poison involved. Before washing your cat, make sure that it is safe for her to get wet, as water may activate some poisons.
2. Always wear nonlatex, disposable gloves. If allowed, wash the animal with large volumes of water. If your pet is having a reaction to a flea product, a mild hand soap or baby shampoo can be used. For oil-based toxins (such as petroleum products), use dishwashing liquid.
3. If the poison is in the eye, flush the eye with large volumes of water or sterile eye wash. (See Administering Eye Medications, page 10.)
4. If the poison is a powder, you will need to dust or vacuum it off.

Inhaled Poisons

Gases, such as carbon monoxide, can cause poisoning.

1. Take your cat into fresh air as quickly as possible.
2. Perform rescue breathing as needed. (See CPR, page 32.)
3. Check for shock. (See Shock, page 103.)

IMPORTANT: To protect your family, including your pet, install a carbon monoxide detector in your home.

Ingested Poisons

It may be appropriate to induce vomiting, but **DO NOT induce vomiting until you speak with a veterinarian or the ASPCA's Animal Poison Control Center.** With some caustic substances, it may be appropriate to give your cat milk to help absorb the poison, but this should be decided on a case-by-case basis. Let your veterinarian or the Animal Poison Control Center advise you.

DO NOT induce vomiting if your cat–

- Is having difficulty breathing.
- Is experiencing seizures, is depressed or is acting unusually excited.
- Is unconscious.
- Has a very slow heart rate. (See Heart Rate and Pulse, page 23.)

Or if–

- The toxin is suspected or known to be a caustic substance (such as a drain opener), an acid (such as from a battery) or a petroleum-based product.
- The object eaten was sharp or pointed.
- The poison container says not to do so.

How to Induce Vomiting

If your veterinarian or the ASPCA's Animal Poison Control Center gives you the okay to induce vomiting, you can give household (3 percent) hydrogen peroxide orally, 1 teaspoon per 10 pounds of body weight. (See Chapter 2: Giving Your Cat Medications, page 9.) Repeat this dosing every 15–20 minutes up to two times, on the way to the veterinary hospital.

Syrup of ipecac can be dangerous to cats and should NOT be used to induce vomiting, unless specifically advised by your veterinarian.

If you are not sure what your pet ate, take the vomit to the hospital with you. If you know what the substance was, take the vomit and the container the toxin was in. **In any case of poisoning, take your pet to the veterinary hospital as soon as possible.**

- If you are unable to induce vomiting, the animal's stomach may need to be pumped.
- If ingestion occurred some time ago and the toxin has already been partially absorbed, blocking further absorption is the next step. This may include giving the pet activated charcoal.
- A few toxic substances have antidotes. To determine an antidote, the veterinarian must know what the animal ate.
- Depending on the poison, there may be serious bodily consequences, including organ failure, and the cat must be treated by a veterinarian with intravenous fluids and medications.

Puncture Wounds and Embedded Object

Puncture wounds can look minor from the outside, but can be deceptively deep and serious. If the wound is not immediately apparent, the injured cat may develop an infection 1 or 2 days after injury.

Signs and Symptoms.

- Bleeding
- Bruising (If this occurs, there may also be significant internal injury to both muscles and organs.)
- Evidence of an embedded object
- Evidence of infection—redness, swelling, discharge, pain
- Small wound in skin. If there are two puncture marks, this is a good indication the wound was caused by a bite. (For how to properly treat a bite wound, see Bite Wounds, page 44, and Venomous Bites and Stings, page 110.)

The Most Common Causes.

Animal abuse, injury from a pointed object

What You Can Do.

1. If the wound is bleeding excessively, control the bleeding. (See Bleeding, page 45.)
2. Check the cat's ABCs; perform CPR as needed. (See CPR, page 32.)
3. Check for shock. (See Shock, page 103.)
4. Administer basic wound care. (See Abrasions, page 38.)
5. If there's an embedded object and it does not appear to penetrate into deep tissues, you can try to remove it with sterilized tweezers, taking care not to push it deeper inside. You should then contact your veterinarian to determine when the wound should be evaluated.
6. If the object appears deeply embedded, do not attempt to remove it. Take the cat to a veterinarian as soon as possible; he may need immediate surgery or intervention once the object is removed.
7. If your cat is ill and has an abscess that has not ruptured, take him to a veterinarian as soon as possible for abscess care.
8. If your cat has an abscess that has ruptured, clean the area as described under Abrasions, page 38, and take him to a veterinarian.

Rectal Prolapse

If your cat strains to defecate and you see a red, sausage-shaped mass pushing out of his anus, he may have rectal prolapse. This is an emergency, so get him to a veterinarian as soon as possible. The earlier it's caught, the better the outcome for your cat.

Signs and Symptoms. Pain; red, sausage-shaped mass out of the anus; straining

The Most Common Causes. Diarrhea; chronic straining to defecate and/or urinate; pushing during whelping (giving birth)

What You Can Do.
1. Lubricate the area with a sterile, water-based lubricant (like K-Y Jelly®).
2. Take your cat to a veterinarian immediately. Depending on the extent of the rectal prolapse, the veterinarian will have to move it back in place and suture the area to make the opening smaller. If the tissue is not viable or healthy, surgery may be needed.

Prevention. If your cat is persistently straining to defecate or has persistent diarrhea, contact your veterinarian to determine the underlying cause and start treatment.

Seizures
As terrifying as they may be to watch, most seizures don't harm your cat. Many have no residual effects at all. But if it's your cat's first seizure, take her to a veterinarian as soon as possible for an evaluation. If it's not your cat's first seizure, but her seizures last longer than 2 minutes or there are multiple, repeating seizures, take her to the veterinarian immediately. This is a medical emergency.

Signs and Symptoms.
Phases of a seizure:

- Before a seizure (*pre-ictal*), your cat may seem dazed or anxious, may seek you or seek a safe place.
- During an active seizure (*ictal*), the animal often will fall over, twitch, urinate, defecate and drool. In addition, she may not recognize you or may fall over and be stiff and rigid (*grand mal seizure*). Some seizures may look like the cat is just staring into space or biting at invisible things (chewing gum seizures).
- After a seizure (*post-ictal*), the animal may be disoriented, walk into walls or appear to be blind. Cats may also behave normally following a seizure.

The Most Common Causes.
Central nervous system causes:

- Abscess
- Epilepsy

First Aid Reference Guide

- Infection in the brain (bacterial, fungal, viral or parasitic)
- Inflammation in the brain
- Malformation of the brain (birth defect)
- Scar tissue in the brain (may occur after a head injury)
- Tumor

Noncentral nervous system causes:

- Glandular disease causing blood sugar to be too low or too high (as may occur in diabetics)
- Low blood calcium
- Organ failure, particularly of the liver and kidney, which are the waste treatment plants of the body (When they malfunction, a large build-up of toxic waste products can occur, causing seizures.)
- Poisoning (such as from certain drugs, plants, lead, heavy metals, antifreeze and chocolate)

The seizure's cause must be identified to determine if it was due to primary respiratory, heart, orthopedic or neurological problems.

What You Can Do.

1. Make sure your cat is in a safe place (not on top of a staircase or anywhere from which a fall is possible).
2. Record how long the active phase of the seizure lasts.
3. Keep a log of your cat's seizures. Include the date, time of day, time after a meal and how long the active seizure phase lasts.
4. Keep your hands away from the animal's mouth. Do not attempt to hold your cat's tongue (the animal will not swallow her tongue). Your cat may not know who you are during a seizure. Many pet owners are bitten while attempting to handle their pets during a seizure.
5. Do not disturb your cat during and after an active seizure.
6. If this is your pet's first seizure, call your veterinarian. Your cat should be examined as soon as possible.
7. Seizures lasting longer than 2 minutes or cluster seizures (seizures repeated one after the other) are medical emergencies; these animals are at risk for very high fevers and brain damage. A veterinarian must immediately examine an animal having cluster seizures.

NOTE: If your cat is placed on anti-seizure medication, understand that the medication does not cure the cause of the seizure; it simply helps to reduce the number or severity of episodes. Your cat will probably have future episodes and require frequent veterinary checkups.

Shock

See also Chapter 5: Respond to a Breathing or Heart Emergency, page 31.

Shock is the body's response to a change in blood flow and oxygen to the internal organs and tissues. This can result from a sudden loss of blood, a traumatic injury, heart failure, severe allergic reaction (anaphylactic shock), organ disease or an infection circulating through the body (septic shock). There are three stages of shock, which may look very different.

Early Shock

The body attempts to compensate for the decreased flow of blood and oxygen to the tissues.

Signs and Symptoms.

- Body temperature that may be low or elevated
- Capillary refill time of 1–2 seconds (See Capillary Refill Time, page 25.)
- Increased heart rate (See Heart Rate and Pulse, page 23.)
- Mucous membranes that are redder than normal (common with septic shock)
- Normal to increased intensity of pulses (may feel like they are pounding)

Middle Stages of Shock

The body begins to have difficulty compensating for the lack of blood flow and oxygen.

Signs and Symptoms.

- Prolonged capillary refill time (See Capillary Refill Time, page 25.)
- Cool limbs
- Depressed mental state
- Increased heart rate (See Heart Rate and Pulse, page 23.)
- Hypothermia (low body temperature of less than 98° F; hairless areas may feel cool to the touch) (See Know What's Normal, page 22.)
- Pale mucous membranes
- Weak pulse

End-Stage or Terminal Shock

This occurs when the body can no longer compensate for the

First Aid Reference Guide

lack of oxygen and blood flow to its vital organs.

Signs and Symptoms.
- Depressed mental state or unconsciousness
- Prolonged capillary refill time (See Capillary Refill Time, page 25.)
- Slow respiratory rate (See Heart Rate and Pulse, page 23.)
- Slow heart rate (See Heart Rate and Pulse, page 23.)
- Weak or absent pulse

IMPORTANT:
Cardiopulmonary arrest may soon follow! Prepare to perform CPR. A cat that is in shock, or that you suspect may be in shock, should be taken to a veterinary hospital immediately.

What You Can Do.
1. Check the cat's ABCs; perform CPR as needed. (See CPR, page 32.)
2. Control bleeding if present. (See Bleeding, page 45.)
3. Warm the animal with a thermal blanket. (See Pet First Aid Kit, page 16.) Wrap the blanket around the animal's body.
4. Elevate the hind end slightly by placing a blanket underneath the hind end.

NOTE: Do not do this if you suspect a broken back. (See Broken Back or Neck, page 57.)
5. Take your cat to a veterinary hospital immediately.

Slipped Disc (Intervertebral Disc Disease)
A slipped disc or intervertebral disc disease is uncommon in cats but can occur when a disc (the cushiony material between each of the vertebrae of the spine) becomes damaged and presses on the adjacent spinal cord. It is most common in the thoracolumbar or lumbar spine. The cause must be determined by an magnetic resonance imaging (MRI) scan or myelogram.

Signs and Symptoms.
- Arched-back stance
- Crying in pain, even without being touched
- Evidence of trauma
- Inability to walk, rear legs that may collapse or show some degree of paralysis, stumbling, dragging of feet or toes
- Lack of control while urinating or defecating
- Not wanting to go up or down stairs

- Trembling
- Very painful back

The Most Common Causes.
Disc injury/trauma

What You Can Do.
1. Take your cat to a veterinarian as soon as possible.
   Carry the animal or restrain
   in a carrier, cage or on a
   board. (See Carrying and
   Transporting Techniques,
   page 29.)
2. If complete paralysis occurs,
   your pet may need surgery
   to walk again.
3. If paralysis is partial, your
   veterinarian may prescribe
   anti-inflammatory medications. Once you give these,
   you must confine your pet in
   a cage or crate because the
   anti-inflammatory medication will make your cat feel
   better and more inclined to
   move around. This could
   potentially worsen his condition. He must be confined to
   a small area for 4 weeks
   (usually longer than the
   medication is given).

Smoke Inhalation

Smoke inhalation is a life-
threatening emergency and
needs veterinary attention
immediately. In fact, smoke can
be more deadly than burns.
Cats that inhale smoke will
gasp or cough and may stop
breathing. Moreover, many
smoke inhalation conse-
quences may not be apparent
for days. So, if your cat is
exposed to fire or smoke, take
her to the veterinarian immediately for an evaluation.

Signs and Symptoms.
- Abnormally fast breathing
  (See Breathing Rate,
  page 23.)
- Cherry-red gums, in the
  case of carbon monoxide
  poisoning
- Coughing
- Discharge from the mouth
  or nose
- Eye discharge
- Labored breathing
- Stopped breathing
- Singed hair with a smoky
  odor on the coat

What You Can Do.
1. **Immediately remove cat
   from smoke and into
   fresh air.**
2. Check the cat's ABCs; perform CPR as needed. (See
   CPR, page 32.)
3. Check for shock. (See
   Shock, page 103.)
4. Take your cat to a veterinary
   hospital immediately.

Some of the life-threatening consequences include—

- Body fluid and electrolyte imbalances.
- Corneal ulcers or damage to the eye surface.
- Fluid accumulation in the lungs or chest cavity.
- Pneumonia.
- Swelling of the mouth and throat.

Sneezing

It is normal for cats to sneeze occasionally. While sneezing itself is not serious, if it is persistent, excessive or accompanied by nasal discharge, it might be a symptom of other health problems that should be addressed by your veterinarian. Depending on the cause, sneezing could be accompanied by a clear, pus-like or bloody nasal discharge.

The Most Common Causes.
- Bleeding disorder (such as a problem with blood clotting)
- Foreign object in the nose or tumor
- Upper respiratory tract infection

An upper respiratory infection can be caused by multiple types of viruses and bacteria. It can lead to sneezing, nasal discharge, ocular discharge, red eyes, fever and anorexia. Your cat may need ophthalmic and/or oral antibiotics and fluids to help her recover.

Strangulation

See also Chapter 5: Respond to a Breathing or Heart Emergency, page 31.

The most common cause of cat strangulation is when the collar gets caught on something or the cat becomes entangled in string or rope. If your cat is strangled, it's important to make sure he's breathing; if he's not, start CPR immediately.

Signs and Symptoms.
Choking, gasping for air

The Most Common Causes.
Abuse, entanglement, collars getting caught on objects

What You Can Do.
1. Check the airway and start CPR, if indicated. (See CPR, page 32.)
2. An animal that becomes strangled or pulls too hard on a leash is at risk for respiratory distress from a fluid buildup in the lungs (non-heart-failure edema), which

can take a few hours to develop.

3. Always take any cat showing signs of strangulation or that has been strangled to a veterinarian as soon as possible.

4. As a preventive measure, always use break-away collars on your cat.

NOTE: You shouldn't use a leash on a cat unless the animal is wearing a harness; a leash should not be attached directly to a cat's collar.

Suffocation

See Head Entrapment, page 79, and Chapter 5: Respond to a Breathing or Heart Emergency, page 31.

Tail Swelling/Injury

While this is not a life-threatening emergency, tail injuries and swelling are common in cats and can be painful.

Signs and Symptoms. Bloody tail, holding tail awkwardly, licking or biting tail

The Most Common Causes. Abscess; burn; wound; trauma (i.e., tail caught in a door, burns from stoves, car accidents, an animal bite)

What You Can Do.

1. Gently examine the area to see if it's red and inflamed. If it is, see Abrasions, page 38, and Bite Wounds, page 44.

2. Take your cat to a veterinarian who may do an x-ray to rule out a fracture. If there is an abscess, antibiotics will be prescribed. If there is a laceration or cut, sutures may be needed. In the case of severe injury, a tail amputation may be needed.

Urinary Accidents/ Incontinence

Your cat may be litter trained, then one day have an accident that leads to several more.

The Most Common Causes.
• Bladder inflammation
• Behavioral problems, stress
• Excessive water consumption
• Glandular disease
• Infection
• Neurological disease
• Steroids like prednisone (These will make the cat urinate more and drink to compensate.)

What You Can Do. Although it's not life threatening, the best thing to do is call your veterinarian as soon as you

First Aid Reference Guide

notice two sequential accidents. The doctor will help determine the cause and possibly prescribe medication.

Urinary Blockage

Urinary blockage is a life-threatening medical emergency and can result from urethral disease, bladder inflammation or a bladder stone. It is most common in adult male cats. If left untreated, the body will begin to reabsorb the waste products normally removed by the urine—this buildup quickly becomes toxic. In addition, the bladder can tear easily after being stretched for prolonged periods and may even rupture. If you suspect a urinary blockage, do not attempt to feel the bladder yourself, as it may be very delicate and may rupture from even the gentlest touch!

Signs and Symptoms.
- Blood in the urine
- Crying, particularly when a cat goes into the litter box
- Coma
- Depression (hiding, unresponsive or refusing food)
- Going in and out of the litter box
- Excessive licking of the genital region
- Long stays in the litter box
- Lethargy
- Loss of appetite
- Slow heart rate
- Squatting to urinate with nothing or only small drops present, and frequent squatting in the same outing
- Swelling of the genital region
- Trying to urinate outside the litter box or in the house
- Vomiting

The Most Common Causes.
Urinary crystals (most common in male cats), urethral mucoid plug, urinary tract stone

What You Can Do.
1. **You must take the animal to a veterinary hospital immediately! This is a medical emergency!**
2. Carry your cat by holding the body behind the back legs so you don't place pressure on the bladder. You can also place your pet in a box or carrier.

At the hospital, with your cat under sedation, a catheter will be placed into the bladder to wash it out and allow the animal to urinate. Some animals need surgery to remove the obstruction or stones, if present.

Prevention.

- Increase water consumption—you can do this by adding water to canned food and putting water fountains around the house (cats love drinking from these).
- Strictly adhere to special diets prescribed for a cat with a history of urinary blockage, bladder infection or stones.
- Always make sure your cat actually passes urine and is not just squatting unproductively.

Finish all antibiotics or other medication prescribed for a urinary tract problem, as the condition may persist for long periods even after your cat seems better.

IMPORTANT: Urethral or urinary obstruction can easily be confused with feline lower urinary tract disease, in which the cat shows very similar signs but is still able to pass urine (not obstructed). This is not life threatening and spontaneously resolves. However, if you are not sure whether your cat is able to pass urine always take him to a veterinarian immediately. Your cat will do much better if the obstruction is caught early.

Vaginal Discharge and Uterine Infection

Unspayed female cats are at risk for uterine infections (pyometra) that can occur at any age. Less common are infections at the site from which the uterus was removed in spayed females.

Signs and Symptoms.

- Discharge from vulva (This may look bloody or may look like pus and have a foul odor. Some uterine infections will not have a discharge due to the cervix being closed.)
- Increased drinking and urination
- Lethargy
- Licking at vulva area
- Loss of appetite
- Vomiting

The Most Common Cause.

Bacterial infection, which causes a build-up of pus in the uterus

What You Can Do. Take your cat to a veterinary hospital immediately. This condition is an emergency and must be dealt with at once, or the uterus may rupture.

Prevention. Spay female cats to reduce the risk of infection.

Venomous Bites and Stings—Snakes, Scorpions and Toads
Snakebites
Poisonous snakes in the United States include—

- **Pit vipers**—These include rattlesnakes, copperheads and cottonmouths. Pit vipers have a depression between their nose and eyes. Their fangs can retract and their heads are triangular in shape.
  - **Rattlesnakes** can be up to 8 feet in length; tails contain a rattle.
  - **Copperheads** are about 4 feet long and have no rattles. The top of the head is a rich, coppery orange color.
  - **Cottonmouths**, also known as water moccasins, can grow to 4 feet in length. The body is dark and the inside of the mouth is snowy white.

- **Coral snakes**—These snakes have fangs that are in the rear of the mouth and are not retractable. They can be up to 3 feet long. They are red, yellow and black in alternating bands.

Signs and Symptoms.
- Bleeding puncture wound
- Blood does not clot
- Breathing stops
- Bruising or sloughing of the skin over the bitten area
- Fang marks may or may not be visible, due to cat hair
- Neurological signs, such as twitching and drooling
- Pain
- Reddening
- Signs of shock
- Swelling of the bitten area; can be severe and progress for more than a day

What You Can Do.
1. If you suspect a poisonous snakebite, attempt to identify the snake, but don't get too close. If you have to kill the snake to protect yourself or your pet, take it with you for identification. **Be aware that the fangs on a decapitated snake's head may be venomous for up to 1½ hours.**

2. Check the cat's ABCs; perform CPR as needed. (See CPR, page 32.)
3. Check for shock. (See Shock, page 103.)
4. Attempt to keep the animal calm and still.
5. Put on nonlatex gloves and wash the wound with water and mild soap. **Do not cut open the wound or attempt to suck out the venom! Do not place ice on the area or use a tourniquet!** (Depending on the situation, such actions may do more harm than good.)
6. Immediately transport your cat to a veterinary hospital.
7. Some non-poisonous snakes may also bite. This bite may cause an allergic reaction. If your pet is bitten by a non-poisonous snake, treat it as you would a puncture wound (see Puncture Wounds and Embedded Objects, page 99, and/or Bite Wounds, page 44) and watch for allergic reactions (see Allergies and Allergic Reactions, page 38). If you are unsure if the snake was poisonous, follow steps 1–6.

Scorpions

Although most scorpion bites are not deadly, being bitten is an emergency, especially since a sting from the more rare bark scorpion can be fatal. Get your cat to a veterinarian immediately if a scorpion sting is suspected.

Signs and Symptoms.
- Accidental urination and defecation
- Breathing problems
- Collapse and potentially death
- Dilated pupils
- Drooling
- Pain
- Paralysis
- Swelling
- Tearing from the eyes

The Most Common Cause. Curiosity

What You Can Do. Take your cat to a veterinarian immediately for treatment.

Toads

The vast majority of toads are not poisonous, but the Colorado River toad (found mainly in the southwestern United States) and the giant brown toad or marine toad (found in Florida, South Texas and Hawaii) can kill a cat. The poisons on a toad's skin can cause severe discomfort and even paralysis or death. So any time you notice the remains of a toad in your cat's mouth or you've seen your cat playing with a toad or its remains, call your veterinarian.

Signs and Symptoms.
- Collapse
- Diarrhea
- Excess salivation
- Fever
- Pawing at the mouth
- Seizures
- Vomiting
- Weakness

The Most Common Causes.
- Licking or eating a toad
- Licking the remnants of where a toad was sitting

What You Can Do.
1. Flush out the cat's mouth with water and look for signs of shock. (See Shock, page 103.)
2. Get your cat to a veterinarian immediately.
3. If it's determined he's been poisoned, it's likely your cat will need to stay overnight at the animal hospital for monitoring with an electrocardiograph and intravenous fluids.

Vomiting

Vomiting can be scary. It can be due to a hairball or it can signal a more serious problem. Your cat will be at risk for dehydration if she vomits multiple times for more than one day and will have to see a veterinarian immediately. On the other hand, if your cat vomits intermittently within the time span of a month or several months and has diarrhea and has lost weight, have her checked by a veterinarian, as it could signal inflammatory bowel disease.

IMPORTANT: Rapid dehydration is possible if the animal is not eating or drinking and is losing body fluids as a result of vomiting and/or diarrhea. Dehydration can lead to shock and death. So pay close attention to your cat's behavior when vomiting.

The Most Common Causes.
- Bacterial, viral or parasitic infection
- Change in diet
- Eating something that cannot pass through the gastrointestinal tract and is stuck, such as a foreign object

- Eating something that upsets the stomach
- Eating toxic materials, including chewing on many types of plants
- Glandular disease (commonly seen in hyperthyroid cats)
- Hairball
- Linear foreign bodies (i.e., string or rope that travels through the stomach and intestines, gets caught, bunches the intestines and saws through the wall of the intestine)
- Motion sickness
- Organ inflammation, infection or failure, such as kidney disease or pancreatitis
- The result of many illnesses

What You Can Do. If your cat is vomiting but otherwise acting normally, then a conservative approach is best. Take the following steps:

1. Give no food or water by mouth for 8–12 hours. Withholding food and water is appropriate only for young adult or otherwise normal, healthy animals. Elderly (over 10 years), very young (under 1 year) or otherwise ill animals should not go without food or water; they should be examined by a veterinarian.
2. If no vomiting occurs while not eating or drinking, offer the animal a small quantity of water and repeat every 2–3 hours as long as vomiting does not recur.
3. If your cat is still not vomiting after 8–12 hours with the water, add a bland or high-fiber diet: ½ teaspoon at a time. Repeat every few hours as long as no vomiting occurs. (See Bland Diet in Diarrhea, page 66.)
4. During the next 48–72 hours, if no vomiting occurs, increase the amount of food and decrease the frequency. During the next 3–5 days, gradually mix the animal's regular diet with the bland diet, slowly returning to a normal dietary regimen.
5. If vomiting occurs despite withholding food and water, or if vomiting occurs on the reintroduction of food and water, you must take the animal to a veterinarian to rule out more serious and possibly life-threatening conditions and to treat dehydration and nausea.

First Aid Reference Guide

6. If other signs of illness accompany the vomiting, such as fever or lethargy, do not withhold food and water. Take the animal directly to a veterinarian for examination.

IMPORTANT: Never let your cat play with string! Balls of yarn (or any other toys that can unravel) are not safe; your pet may accidentally ingest the string or yarn. If you see a string exiting the anus do not pull the string as this may tear the intestines. But if it is in the mouth and you can see the entire string, try pulling gently. If there's any resistance or your cat is in pain, stop and take him to a veterinary hospital as soon as possible.

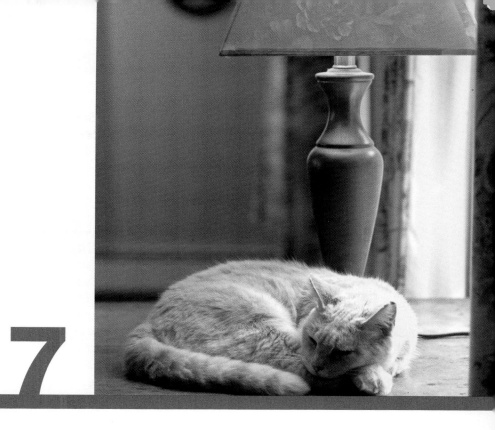

7

When It's Time to Say Goodbye

Chances are you regard your cat as a furry family member. So saying goodbye is certainly not easy. But sometimes, no matter how hard you try, it's just not possible to keep your cat happy and well any longer. Perhaps he is old and in failing health; or he may be young but afflicted with a painful, chronic condition that will worsen over time; or perhaps he was involved in a traumatic accident.

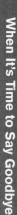

Euthanasia

When your gut starts telling you, "It is time," talk to your veterinarian about the appropriate next step. Many times, euthanasia is the only humane option. In this procedure, your veterinarian will give your cat an overdose of anesthesia or barbiturate that will relax her and bring about a quick and painless death.

Ask your veterinarian about the best time of day to do this. Often when veterinary clinics are the least busy—usually during the first appointment in the morning or the last one at night—they can provide the most privacy. Or you might be able to arrange for the veterinarian to come to your house to do the procedure.

You will also have to choose whether or not you want to be present. Keep in mind that it might upset your cat to see you extremely distraught.

You also will have to decide what to do with your cat's remains. Your cat can be cremated with other animals or cremated individually, in which case her ashes can be returned to you. Or you may choose to bury your cat in a pet cemetery or—if permitted by local zoning laws—in your backyard.

Bereavement Support and Counseling

Losing your cat is similar to losing any other family member, so give yourself permission to grieve and seek support if you're not feeling better in a few weeks. There are many pet bereavement and support groups, so don't hesitate to ask your veterinarian for suggestions.

Here are some resources you may find helpful:

- The American Society for the Prevention of Cruelty to Animals' (ASPCA) Pet Loss Hotline: 800-946-4646 (Enter the PIN number 140-7211 and then add your own phone number; you will be contacted by an ASPCA counselor.)
- The Association of Pet Loss and Bereavement: *www.aplb.org*
- Your state's veterinary school for information on local support groups

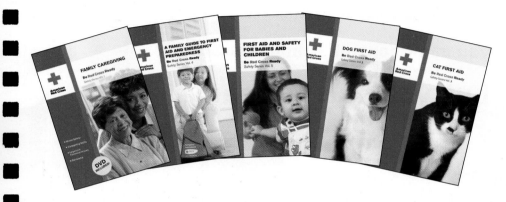
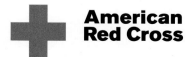

you can't stop a hurricane.

you can't predict an earthquake.

you can't control a thunderstorm.

but you can be ready.

Visit www.redcross.org

Check out our interactive **Be Red Cross Ready** presentation, then visit *www.redcross.org/store* to find a variety of products and resources to help you be more prepared.

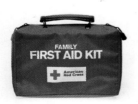

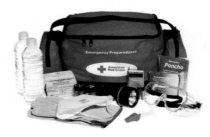

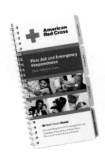

Be Red Cross Ready

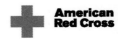

H20344